Aortic Dissection:
The Patient Guide

Acknowledgements

Aortic Dissection Awareness UK & Ireland would like to thank all of the patients and family members who contributed to this Guide, and the healthcare professionals who helped us develop it.

Specific acknowledgements are due to:

Aortic Dissection Awareness patient contributors and reviewers:

Dan Burgess, Matt Consadine, Robert Denton, Moira Dick, Cliff Grover, Simon Jones, Rachel Knight, Mark Lewis, Prashant Navaratnarajah, Gareth Owens, Llyr Rees, Alison Roberts-Pagent, Lisa Skinner, John Tiernan, Keith Watson, Richard Westray, Alex Williams.

Endorsements:

Mr. Simon Kendall, President, on behalf of the Society for Cardiothoracic Surgery in Great Britain & Ireland

Mr. Jonathan Boyle, President, on behalf of the Vascular Society for Great Britain & Ireland

Concept and co-ordinating Editor:
Cliff Grover

Illustrations and Graphic Design:
madebytwo.co.uk

Clinical Review team:

- Miss Ana Lopez-Marco, Consultant Cardiac and Aortic Surgeon, Barts Heart Centre
- Mrs Emma Hope, Aortic Specialist Nurse and Nurse Case Manager to Mr Geoff Tsang, Cardiothoracic Dept., University Hospital Southampton NHS Foundation Trust
- Prof Rob Sayers, Consultant Vascular Surgeon & George Davies Chair of Vascular Surgery, University of Leicester. Medical Advisor to Aortic Dissection Awareness UK & Ireland
- Dr Stephanie Curtis, Consultant Cardiologist in Adult Congenital Heart Disease, Inherited Cardiac Conditions and Obstetric Cardiology, Bristol Heart Institute
- Dr Hannah Mustard, Specialist Clinical Psychologist, Adult Congenital Heart Disease, Bristol Heart Institute
- Dr Sue Potter, General Practitioner, Moss Grove Surgery, Kingswinford, West Midlands.
- Ms Kathryn Hewitt, Advanced Clinical Practitioner - Cardiac Surgery, University Hospitals Birmingham NHS Foundation Trust

Copyright:

Table of contents

Part B - Back Home: Life After Aortic Dissection

Part C - For Family and Carers

Foreword

Most people go through their lives knowing nothing about aortic dissection. You are one of a small, special group of survivors of this rare, life-threatening condition which I joined in 2016.

Welcome!

This Guide has been put together by patients, family and carers, for patients, family and carers. It contains everything we wish we had known when we were in your position, during your initial recovery. I suggest you use the table of contents and dip in at first to the topics you are interested in. Let your partner, family or carer read this Guide too, so that they can better understand and help you – and themselves.

I would like to thank the team of patients, family, carers and healthcare professionals who have spent a year working on Aortic Dissection: The Patient Guide. I know it will help you a lot. The national patient association for aortic dissection, which I chair, also offers great friendship and support to patients and relatives. Membership is FREE, and you will find our contact details in the Guide. We would love for you to join us whenever you feel ready.

I wish you good luck with your personal aortic dissection journey. You are not alone. Aortic Dissection Awareness UK & Ireland is here to help. Remember, as an aortic dissection survivor you have already beaten the odds, so Today Is a Good Day!

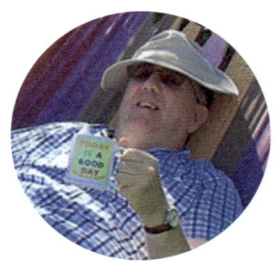

Gareth Owens

Chair, Aortic Dissection Awareness UK & Ireland

"
You are not alone.
Aortic Dissection Awareness
UK & Ireland is here to help.
Remember, as an aortic
dissection survivor you have
already beaten the odds, so
Today Is a Good Day!

About this Guide

Aortic Dissection: The Patient Guide covers what you and your family need to know after you have had an aortic dissection. You may have been given it in hospital or found it on the internet.

The Guide is in three parts.

Part A - Early Days

Read this first. It tells you what you need to know in the days and weeks immediately following your aortic dissection.

Part B - Back Home: Life After Aortic Dissection

This part will help you understand how to adjust to your aortic dissection once you are back home.

Part C - For Family and Carers

This section covers how family and carers can help, and what you and your family need to understand for the long term.

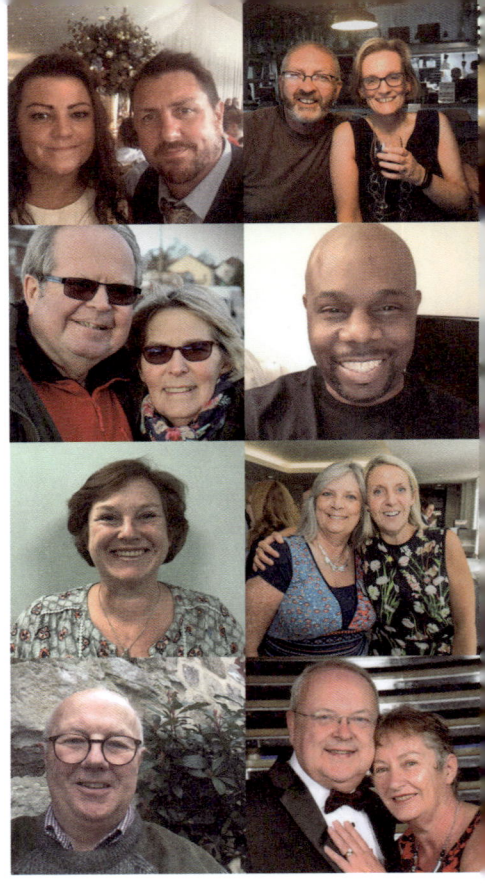

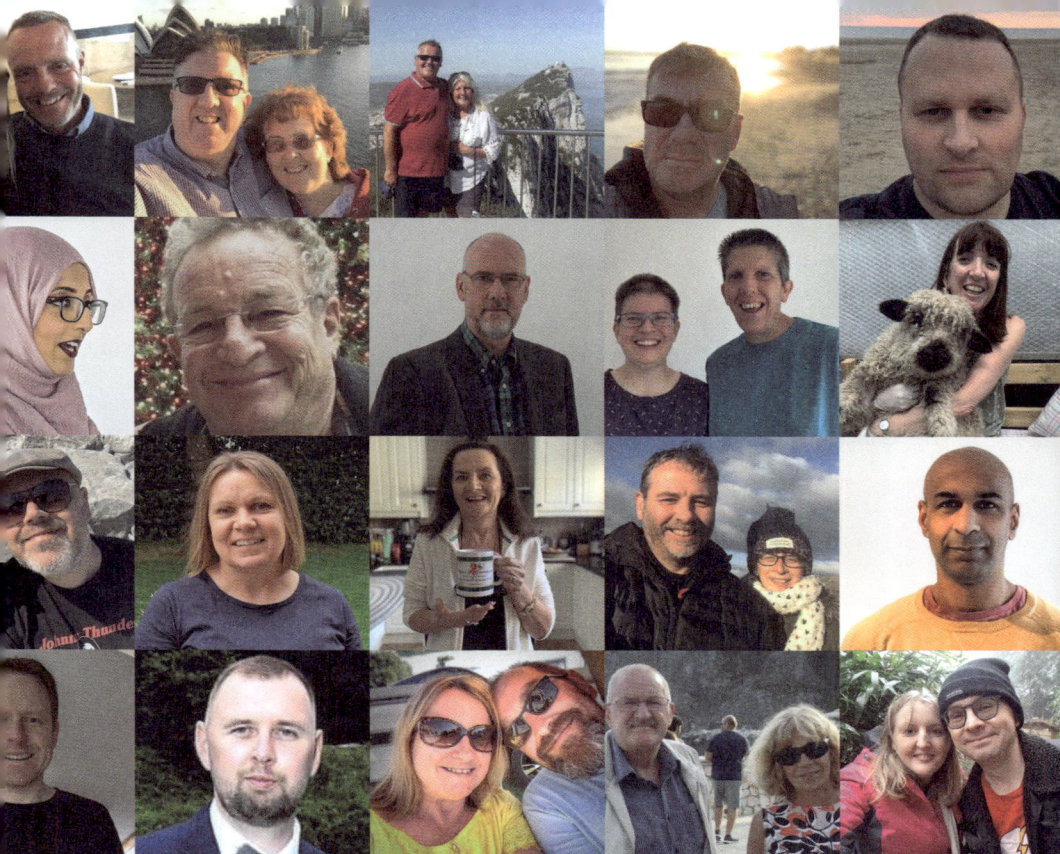

These are some of our members who have recovered from an aortic dissection.

Your aortic dissection may not be identical to the experiences of other patients. Events, treatments and recoveries differ depending upon the nature and type of your dissection, how you were treated and your personal health and circumstances. This Guide aims to cover the most important things you should know, but parts of it may not apply to you. Read the parts that are most relevant to you, at the appropriate time.

For your family and friends, having a loved one suffer an aortic dissection can be a worrying time. It is important for them to understand what happened and how they can help you and help themselves. Part C of the Guide includes information specifically for family, carers and friends. They should also read the section titled 'What is an aortic dissection?', which comes next.

Part A

Early Days

- In Hospital
- Ycur Discharge and Early Recovery

In Hospital

What is an aortic dissection? – the basics

Aortic dissection (AD) is a serious condition that affects the aorta. The aorta is the main artery from your heart and feeds blood to every part of your body, including the heart itself, the head and brain, arms, legs and vital organs in the chest and belly.

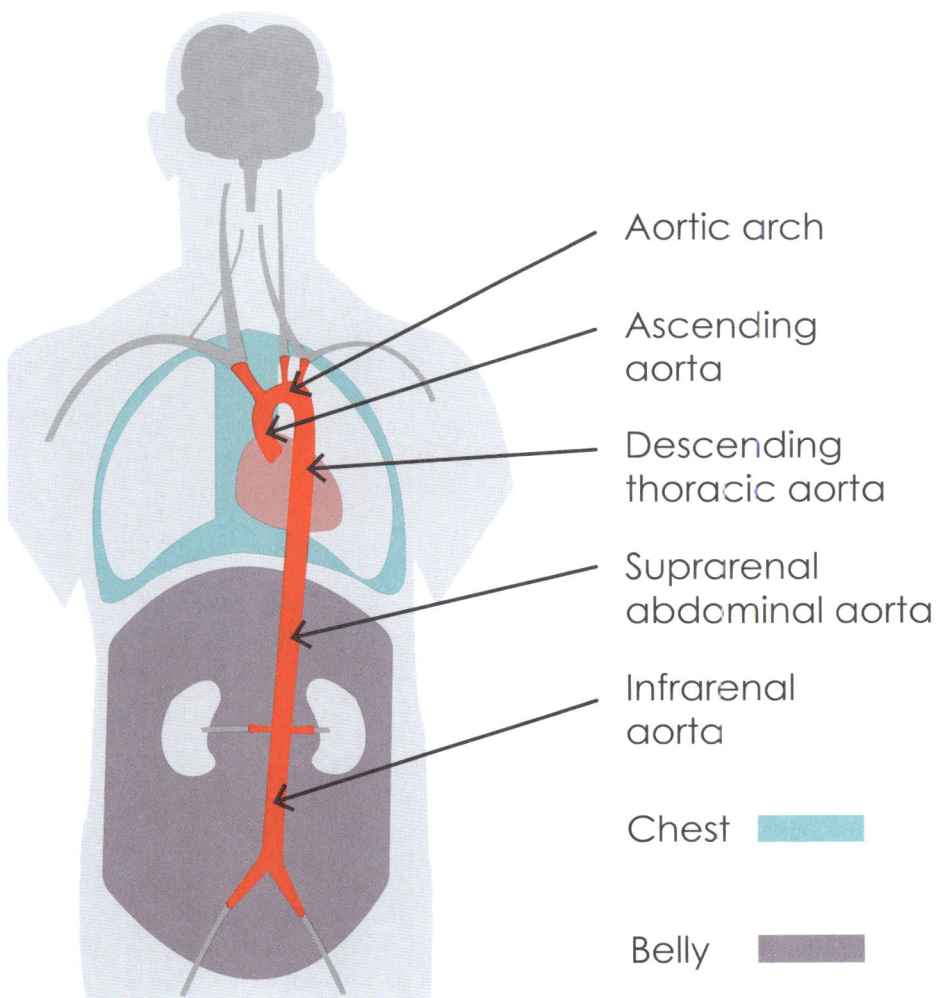

Aortic arch

Ascending aorta

Descending thoracic aorta

Suprarenal abdominal aorta

Infrarenal aorta

Chest

Belly

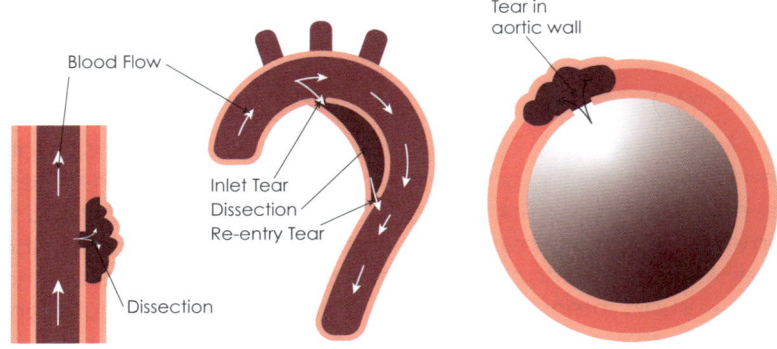

Blood Flow

Inlet Tear
Dissection
Re-entry Tear

Dissection

Tear in
aortic wall

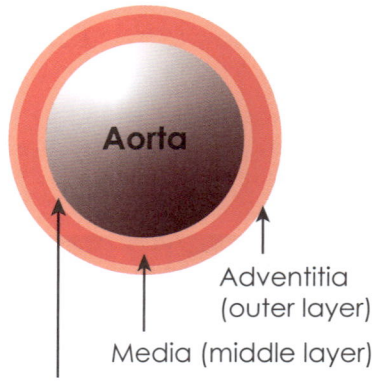

Aorta

Aortic dissection

An aortic dissection starts when there is a tear in the inner layer of your aorta. The wall of the aorta is made up of three layers: inner, middle and outer.

The inner layer is thin and provides a smooth surface for blood to flow past. It also provides a seal between the flowing blood and the middle layer.

The middle layer is thicker and is made up of elastic muscle fibres, which give the aorta the strength to withstand the pressure of your blood as it flows past (your blood pressure).

The outer layer is thin, like the inner layer. It contains and seals the middle layer and gives structure and support for the aorta.

You may also hear the layers of the aorta being referred to by their medical names: the intima, media and adventitia, respectively.

Adventitia
(outer layer)

Media (middle layer)

Intima (inner layer)

Layers of the wall of the aorta

If the inner layer of the aorta develops a tear, this allows blood to circulate between the inner and the middle layer, creating two separate channels of circulating blood instead of one, hence the word dissection. The original channel is called the true lumen and the new channel opened by the tear is called the false lumen.

When the aorta dissects it will generally also swell to a larger diameter. Often, blood flowing in the false lumen will find its way back into the true lumen at another tear in the inner layer which develops further along.

When the aorta tears, it is usually very painful and the pain is usually sudden and intense. The pain may occur anywhere from the chest area up towards the head, neck and jaw, down the back and/or into the abdomen. It may also travel to the arms or legs. In some cases, the pain can feel like a heart attack. You can also lose consciousness. Although the pain is usually intense to start with, it can also move around and even subside, and a minority of dissections cause very little pain.

When the aorta tears like this, it is extremely serious. The dissection may disrupt blood flow to the heart, brain, limbs, organs or any part of the body, which will also then be affected.

The initial tear in the inner layer can occur from just above the heart, or anywhere along the entire length of the aorta, to near the top of the legs.

> An aortic dissection is categorised according to where the initial tear in the lining occurs, as this also helps to guide your subsequent treatment.

Type A

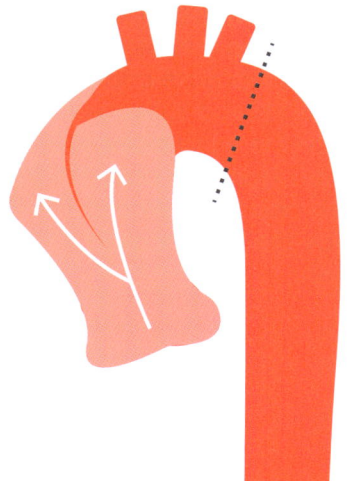

Type B

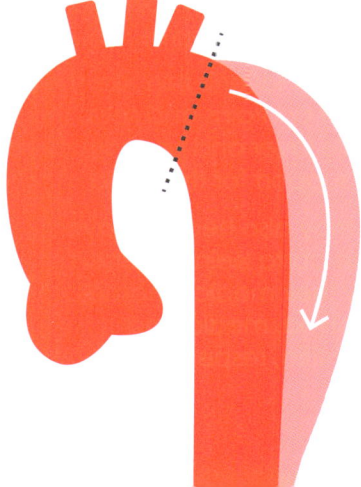

Type A dissection

If the tear in the lining is in the first part of the aorta near where it exits the heart, or in the arch, this is called a Type A dissection.

A Type A dissection can cause a number of serious and time-critical problems, such as a heart attack, blood to collect around the heart, or loss of blood and therefore oxygen to the brain. This is a surgical emergency: correct diagnosis and treatment within hours is crucial. Most Type A dissection patients have immediate emergency surgery with a specialist heart surgeon to repair their aorta. This involves opening the chest, removing the diseased part of the aorta and replacing it with an artificial graft. If the aortic valve (where the blood leaves the heart) is affected it may be possible to repair the valve but it often has to be replaced.

Example Type A ascending aorta repair (including 'hemi-arch'), no valve replacement

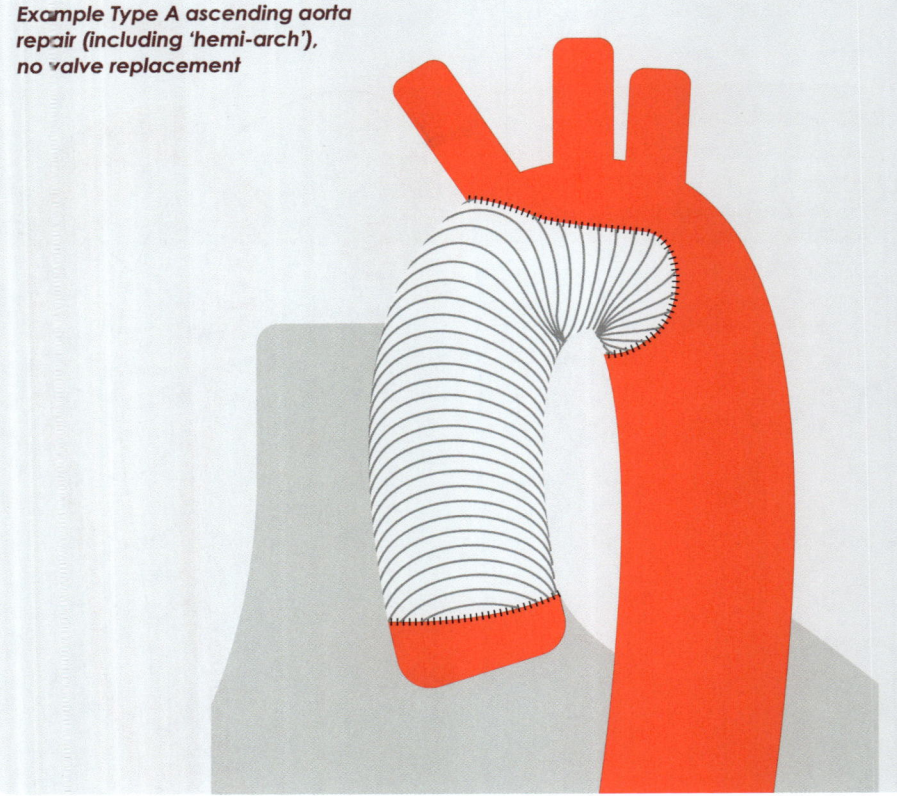

When a Type A dissection also involves the aortic arch, special surgery is needed. The arch feeds blood to the brain and that supply must be preserved in order to protect the brain during the surgery. This surgery is usually only available in major aortic centres.

One of the repair options can be seen below, where the entire aortic arch has been replaced and the initial part of the descending aorta stabilised with a stent called a 'Frozen Elephant Trunk'.

Example complex Type A repair
- arch replacement and Frozen
Elephant Trunk ('FET')

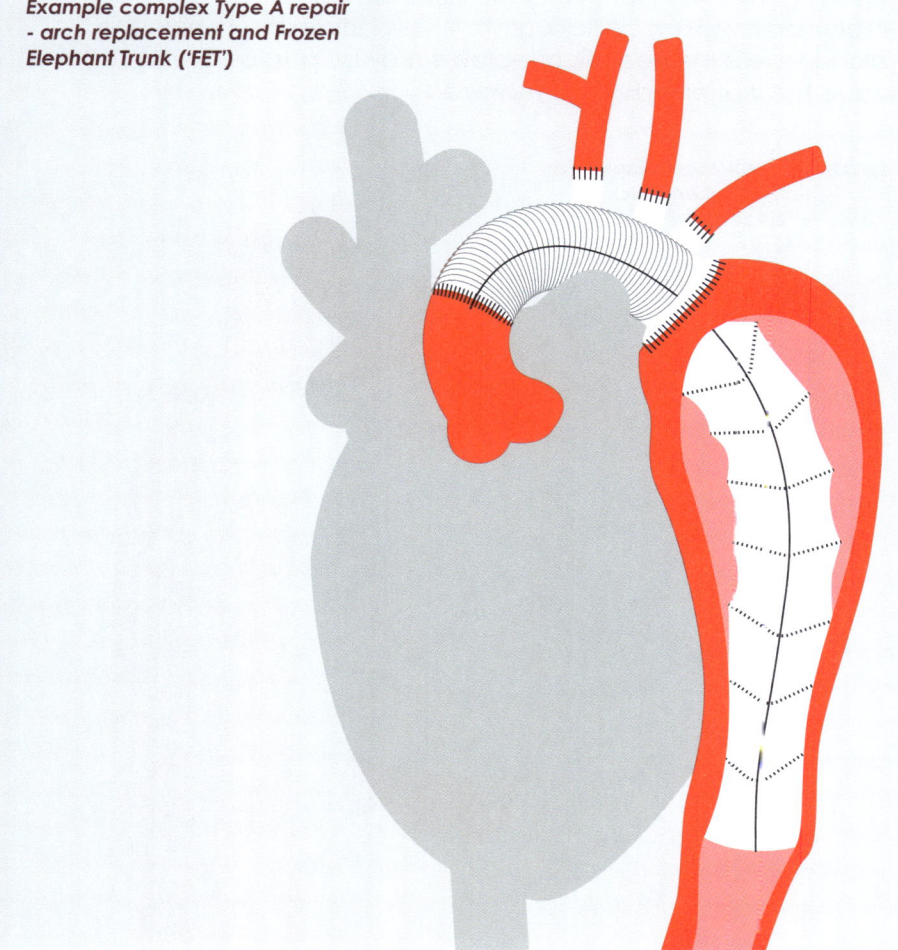

Type B dissection

If the tear is in the descending part of the aorta, beyond where the artery that goes down the left arm branches off, this is called a Type B dissection. Type B dissection can cause complications due to a loss of blood flow to one or more major organs of the body. However, the blood flow to the heart and brain is typically not affected and, depending on how severe the loss of blood flow is, most vital organs have some capacity to operate with a reduced blood supply. Usually, there is more time to decide on the appropriate course of treatment in Type B dissection.

Around 70% of Type B dissections are managed medically by controlling blood pressure to a safe level, followed by long-term monitoring.

More complicated Type B dissections often require surgery to replace the affected section of the aorta. As an alternative, and when suitable, a minimally-invasive repair can be done using a 'stent' inserted via an artery in the groin – this is called an endovascular repair; TEVAR or EVAR for short. A TEVAR is an endovascular repair limited to the thoracic (T) region, i.e. your chest. EVAR is a term for a general endovascular repair, or a repair below the thoracic region – some dissections extend as far as the arteries at the top of your legs.

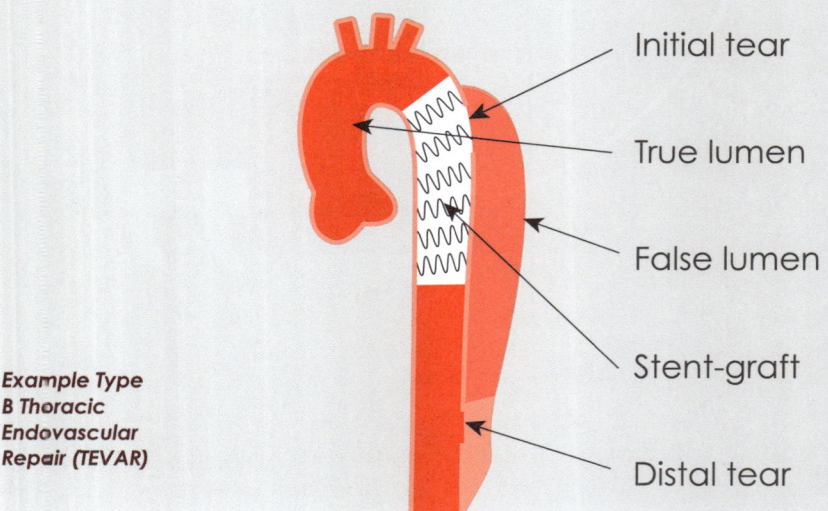

Initial tear

True lumen

False lumen

Stent-graft

Distal tear

Example Type B Thoracic Endovascular Repair (TEVAR)

"

My type B aortic
dissection occurred
in March 2003. It has been
challenging, but with a positive
attitude I have been able to greet
each and every morning since with
a smile and these five words:

"TODAY IS A GOOD DAY"

*Dan Burgess, founder of
Aortic Dissection Awareness
UK and Ireland*

"

What happened in my case?

When you feel ready for it, your medical team should provide you with as much information as you would like regarding your specific case.

The key questions you should ask early on include:

- what happened to me?
- which part of my aorta was affected by my dissection?
- did I have surgery to repair my aorta? Was it open surgery or endovascular surgery? Or am I being 'medically managed'
- can I have a sketch of what happened and any repair?
- did I have any complications?
- do I have any dissection or other disease in other parts of my aorta that might give me a problem or need to be repaired in the future?

The pages at the back of this Guide are for you and your medical team to use to help you understand your particular case. They include blank pages where your team can draw 'before' and 'after' sketches of your aorta and a longer list of possible questions, with space for the answers. See pages 94-95.

Why did I have an aortic dissection?

Aortic dissection is a rare condition, affecting around six people per year per 100,000 head of population; around 60% of these are Type A.

Aortic dissection has a number of underlying causes, not all of which are fully understood. However, they all have a common feature which is that the aortic wall has become weak and unable to withstand the pressure of your blood, or the movement of the aorta created by the heart beating and your body moving.

There are various risk factors for aortic dissection, including general health risk factors and genetic risk factors. No direct relationship exists which covers every case, hence the term 'risk factors'. The more risk factors that someone has, or the more extreme a factor is, the more likely they are to have a dissection.

These risk factors are discussed in the next few pages.

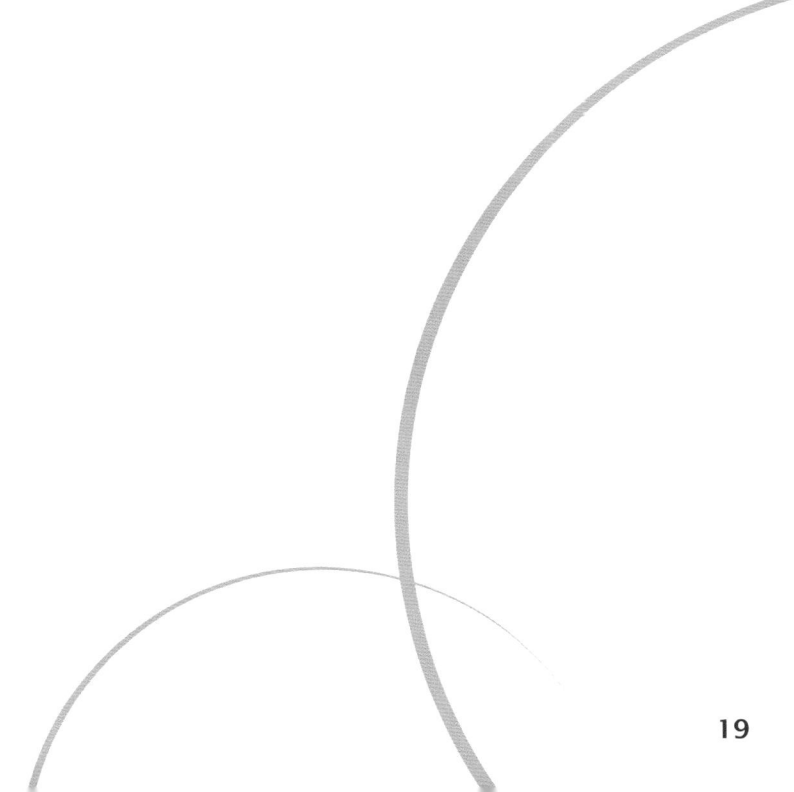

General risk factors

Some general factors can predispose someone to an aortic dissection.

- **Aneurysm** – a bulge in the aorta (which may be genetic, as with aortic dissection itself). These are more common with advancing age.
- **High blood pressure** – high blood pressure directly exerts excessive force on the aorta, forcing it to stretch.
- **Bicuspid aortic valve (BAV)** – the aortic valve is found between the heart and aorta. It opens to let the blood out and then closes to stop blood leaking back into the heart. BAV is when the aortic valve, which normally has three leaflets ('tricuspid'), has only two leaflets ('bicuspid'). This can cause the valve to leak or become narrow. A 'murmur' may be heard through a stethoscope if this is the case, which is the sound of blood flowing backwards through the valve after it has closed.

  BAV affects 1-2% of the population. The risk of aortic dissection with a BAV is difficult to quantify and research on this is ongoing. However, AD patients with BAV tend to be younger than those with a tricuspid valve, are less likely to have high blood pressure and may have other aortic disease prior to dissection (either undiagnosed or diagnosed).
- **Trauma** – trauma such as a car crash can cause an aortic dissection, though normally only if the aorta already has some weakness. For severe trauma such as this, the aorta can also rupture.
- **Illegal/illicit drugs** – cocaine usage is a known risk factor for aortic dissection.

- **Atherosclerosis** – in a similar way to building up plaque (fatty deposits) inside a person's coronary arteries, plaque can build up on the inside of the aorta and accelerate degradation of the aortic tissues. Plaque is often due to risk factors such as smoking, diabetes, high blood pressure and high cholesterol.

  A particular risk is that of a 'penetrating atherosclerotic ulcer' or PAU. This is an ulcer which usually forms beneath plaque and penetrates into the aortic wall, causing a weak spot in the wall. This can (but may not) initiate an aortic dissection. Up to 7% of aortic dissections are due to a PAU.

- **Weight lifting and other sports** – weight lifting can induce extreme blood pressure peaks, particularly if the person does not breathe properly or holds their breath. On its own, weight lifting should not cause an aortic dissection but can precipitate one if there is already an aortic weakness.

  A minority of dissections are precipitated by other sports, including contact sports, typically involving elevated blood pressure, heavy contact, turning or stretching. Again, such activities should not cause an aortic dissection but can initiate one if there is an aortic weakness.

- **Pregnancy** – pregnancy is also a risk factor for aortic dissection. Carrying a baby increases stress on the mother's cardiovascular system and causes hormonal changes. Some of the drugs that are used around the time of delivery can also increase the risk. High blood pressure in pregnancy or pre-eclampsia will increase this risk.

Genetic risk factors

In addition to the general risk factors, aortic disease and dissection can run in families and hence can be called 'familial' or 'heritable' (inherited) conditions. In these cases, the disease is caused by faulty genetic mutations. Mutations are very small changes in the genetic makeup of cells which make up our bodies, and can lead to changes in the cell and tissue properties. Mutations are sometimes called variants. When these mutations affect the aorta, they fall into one of two categories.

- **Syndromic** – 'syndromic' means that the patient will usually have a number of typical features together, i.e. a syndrome. These can include tall stature, long limbs, curvature of the spine, a particular facial appearance, or 'tortuous' blood vessels. Not everyone with a syndrome will display all of these.

The most common syndromes are Marfan, Loeys-Dietz, and Ehlers-Danlos Syndromes. Turner's Syndrome is another condition, which is confined to women. It can lead to bicuspid aortic valve and aortic dissection. Turner's syndrome is often associated with short stature and other features (see NHS websites).

All of these syndromes are sometimes referred to as 'connective tissue disorders' or CTDs, as it is the connective tissues of the body that are affected, leading to the features listed. As well as the syndromic features noted, all these genetic disorders also typically weaken the aortic tissues and predispose a person to aortic dissection.

Overall, somewhere between 5% and 20% of aortic dissections are associated with CTDs. Aortic dissections due to CTDs tend to occur at an earlier age (typically age 40-50) than for other types. Where a patient has one of these syndromes, the culprit gene can usually be identified.

- **Non-Syndromic –** in non-syndromic cases the condition runs in the family but there are none of the other physical features described in the syndromes above. Though these cases clearly have a genetic basis which can sometimes be identified through testing, it may not be possible to find a culprit gene in every case.

In both groups, the faulty genetic mutation is usually inherited and when that is so, it occurs in such a way that parents have a 50:50 chance of passing it on to each of their children. It affects males and females equally and does not skip a generation. However, some members of the family may be more severely affected than others. In a very small minority of cases, the person affected will not have inherited the condition from anyone, but will be the start of a family trait.

If you have had an aortic dissection, it is important to consider whether you should undergo testing to see if you have any known genes which contributed to your dissection. This is particularly relevant to those dissecting before they are 60 years old.

If your aortic dissection is found to be due to a genetic cause this may also involve your family. Genetic testing is covered in more detail (see pages 83-87) where you can read about how genetic testing is done, both for yourself and your family.

How should I be cared for in hospital?

After your aortic dissection, your progress through the hospital will depend on what type of dissection you had, how serious it was, whether you had surgery or not, and any complications. Generally, your care will start in a high-intensity ward and progress to an ordinary ward until you are discharged. Your treatment route will also depend on the particular facilities your hospital has.

Many aortic dissection patients are cared for first in an Intensive Care Unit (ICU), sometimes known as an Intensive Therapy Unit (ITU). From there they are moved to a High Dependency Unit (HDU) or a Coronary Care Unit (CCU). As they improve, they are transferred to an ordinary cardiac, vascular or surgical ward prior to discharge home. Occasionally, complications such as a stroke or spinal cord injury mean that patients are transferred to a specialist unit before they can go home.

While there may be differences in recovery, what all patients have in common is that the most important aspects of recovery are rest, sleep, nutrition and recovering their mobility. The hospital will monitor how you are managing with these and will do everything to ensure you are progressing well. You will have 'observations' taken every few hours, such as blood pressure, temperature, heart rate, blood oxygen level and your fluid intake and output. These are entirely normal and nothing to be worried about. You will probably be connected to various monitors to start with and these will be gradually disconnected as your recovery progresses.

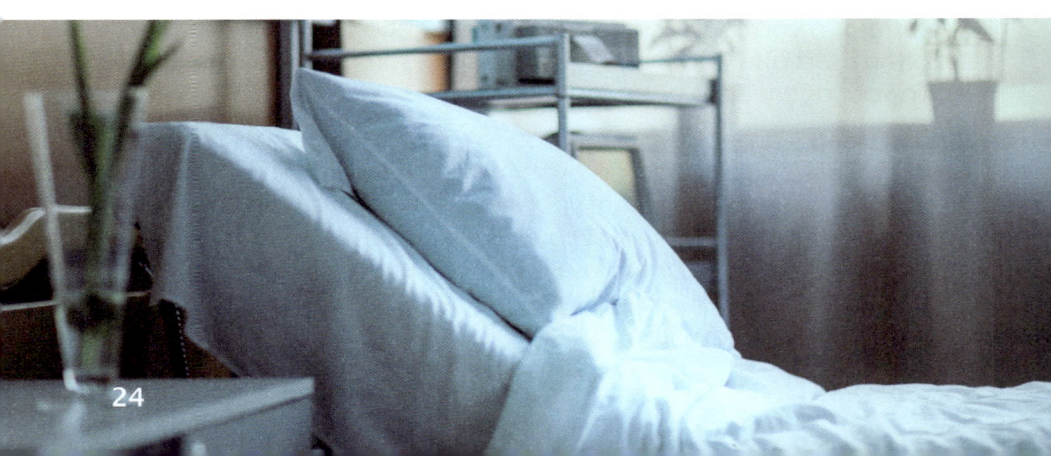

What medicines will I be given?

While you are in hospital, you will probably receive one or more medications. These will be given to you by the nursing staff after they are prescribed by your doctors. You may not be completely aware of what medications you are given and there may be a number of them. They will have been chosen to be appropriate to your specific case.

- **For pain** – a range of medications can be given including paracetamol or stronger medications such as morphine or fentanyl. These may initially be injected into a vein via a 'drip'. As you recover and the pain subsides, these will change to pain relief tablets.

- **Sedatives** – especially if you have had complex surgery, you may be kept asleep with sedatives and on a breathing machine for a while – this is what is known as an induced coma. Sedation will be withdrawn when you are ready, but it is not uncommon to need several attempts before sedation can be fully withdrawn.

- **Blood pressure medication** – may be given to you to control your blood pressure and avoid putting too much pressure on your aorta. This may be pills (often beta blockers), and/or initially, via a drip into one of your veins. Effective blood pressure control is crucial, especially when managing a Type B dissection.

- **Anticoagulants** (sometimes called 'blood thinners') – if you have had your aortic valve replaced during surgery with a mechanical valve, you will be given warfarin to prevent your blood from clotting on the valve and affecting its operation. You may be given a different anticoagulant if you have not had a mechanical valve replacement but have experienced atrial fibrillation, or to reduce the risk or effects of a stroke.

- **Statin** – a statin is a medication that reduces the build-up of cholesterol in your arteries and protects your heart for the long term. It is often used after a dissection, especially if some degree of plaque within your arteries has been found.

- **Help to sleep** – especially as you start to recover, a busy hospital ward can be a noisy place and you may experience difficulty sleeping. Sleep is a vital part of your recovery, so if you are having trouble sleeping, you can ask if you can take a sleeping tablet. Alternatively, you could try to use a pair of well-fitting headphones or earbuds and play some soothing music or 'white noise' such as the sound of rain - perhaps from a white noise App on your phone.

What special help might I need after surgery?

If you have had surgery for either a Type A or Type B dissection, you may need special help, which your medical staff will recognise and provide. These issues are less likely in medically-managed Type B dissection cases.

Not everyone will experience these problems, but the following types of help are common for some aortic dissection patients.

- **Help to breathe** – often, especially with an open-chest operation, your lungs may have been affected so that you cannot breathe as normally and easily as you used to. This will recover in a short time, but you may be given a breathing mask or a nasal oxygen supply to help in the interim.

- **Chest drainage tubes** – if you have had surgery, it is common for chest drain tubes to be placed. These allow any build-up of fluids inside your chest cavity in the days after your surgery to be monitored and drained. The chest drains will be removed at the right time once your medical staff are happy it is safe to do so.

- **Nutrition and blood tests** – your blood will be regularly tested and checked for the necessary components, and to ensure everything in your body is working correctly, especially your kidneys. You can expect regular blood samples to be taken, probably every day at first. The hospital should give you appropriate meal selections and may also give you supplements to help you recover.

- **Feeding** – if you spent over a week in ICU, it is possible that you will have been given your nutrition through a feeding tube inserted into your stomach via your nose. This will be removed once you are able to swallow safely and eat enough calories. At this stage, you may find the taste of normal food unappealing, but your normal sense of taste will return in time.

- **Speech** – some surgical procedures, including the use of a tracheostomy tube (used for severe breathing or lung difficulties), may affect your ability to speak clearly. Your medical staff will observe how well you are able to talk and help you understand and manage your particular situation. You may be provided with one or more visual aids to help you make yourself understood. Speech difficulties should only be temporary and resolve in a few days or weeks, but sometimes, voice difficulties persist after you are out of hospital (see page 52).

26

- **Help with going to the toilet** – in the first few days, you may have a urinary catheter to measure how much urine you are passing. It will be removed a few days after surgery, once the medical staff are happy that your kidneys are working well and you are passing enough urine. If you are unable to get out of bed once the catheter has been removed, you will get help with going to the toilet. This will be necessary only until you can manage by yourself.

- **Strange dreams and fears** – a side-effect of anaesthesia, surgery, and some medications is that you may get strange dreams, hallucinations or nightmares. They may feel very real. This is normal and is due to the procedures and medications, not your own state of mind. You might also become fearful of what has happened to you and how you are being looked after. You may even be worried about what people are doing to you and whether you are getting the right treatment. Some of these things will be noticeable to your family.

  Such experiences are often called 'ICU delirium'. This is a recognised side effect of the trauma you have been through and the medications you need to help you recover. These experiences will eventually decrease and disappear as you recover and the medications are reduced and eventually stopped. You and your family can rest assured that this is normal, that your dreams and hallucinations are not real and that you are in fact being treated properly and professionally by the medical staff.

> If you have these experiences and are worried, talk to your nursing staff on the ward.

- **Heart rhythm disturbances** (arrhythmia) – especially after major cardiothoracic surgery, your heart may not beat normally and regularly. Around one third of patients who have surgery for aortic dissection develop atrial fibrillation, where the heart beats irregularly and sometimes very fast. This can feel strange and disconcerting. It is often treated with medications to help the heart go back to a normal rhythm and to minimise the risk of a stroke. Sometimes, the irregular heart rhythm may persist when you get home and you will need to continue taking medication for it until your heart goes back to its normal rhythm.

27

- **Stroke** – sometimes, patients who have an aortic dissection will also experience a stroke, either when their dissection happens, during surgery, or afterwards. A stroke can lead to difficulties with speech or movement. If you have had a stroke, you will be specially monitored for its effects and referred to a stroke specialist or stroke unit to help you get over the effects. For more information see the section on complications on page 51.

- **Spinal cord injury** – aortic dissection and surgery can sometimes affect your spinal cord and cause a partial or total loss of sensation in your lower body and legs. This is often temporary; rarely will it be permanent. Your medical team will assess you for any spinal cord injury and will ensure that you get the right specialist help if you are affected.

> If you are worried at all by any of the things described on pages 26-28, let a nurse know and they will ensure that you get the right help and information.

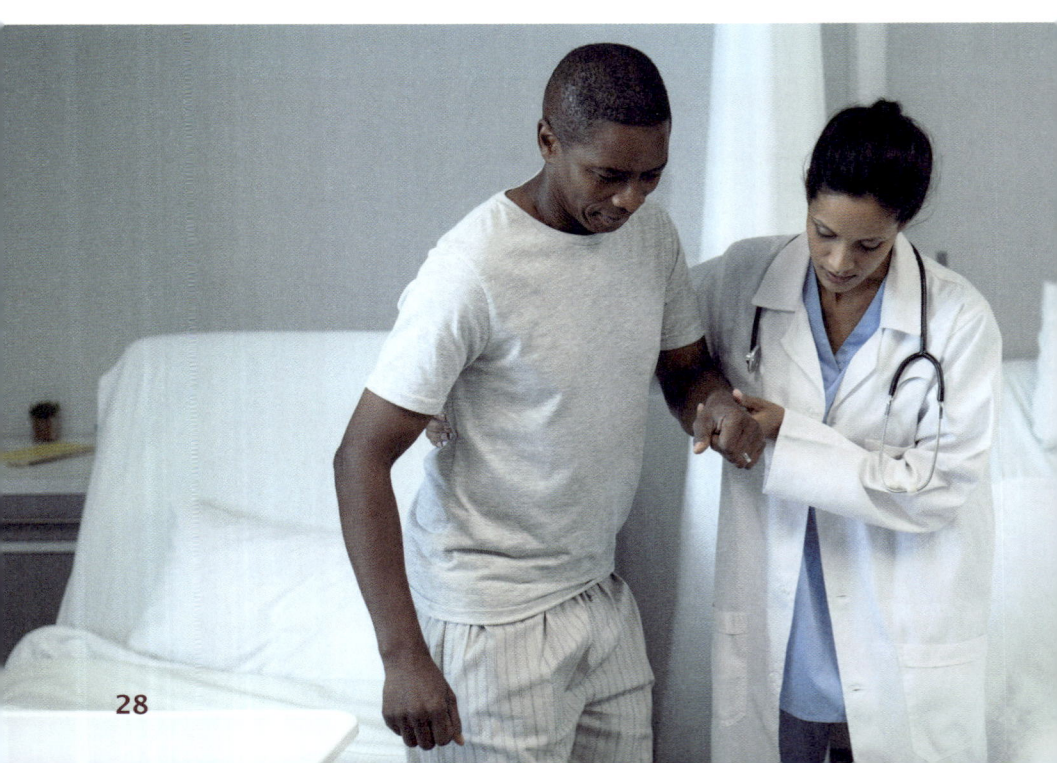

What physical rehabilitation can I expect in hospital?

You should get help from a physiotherapist to get moving again. At first, you may find you need to use a walking frame or a walking stick to help you and to ensure you are safe when on your feet. Take advantage of this help if it is offered. You will be able to dispense with the walking aids as you get stronger. You may also be given breathing exercises to help your lungs recover. Make sure you do the exercises your physiotherapist prescribes. They will make you stronger.

As your walking improves, the physiotherapist will check that you can safely go up and down stairs. This usually happens shortly before you go home. Your physiotherapist should also check whether you need any walking aids at home. You may also be seen by an occupational therapist to see whether you need any other assistance to resume your normal daily life. There is more on this in the next section.

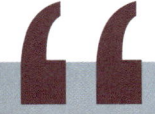

One of the highlights of my stay in hospital was the first time I walked around the ward. I had help from nurses, but I could also hear other patients shouting encouragement from their beds. It was so good to hear the support from fellow patients. Eventually it was time to go home.

Matt Consadine

Your Discharge And Early Recovery

Before you are discharged from hospital, a member of the nursing staff should discuss your discharge arrangements and answer any questions you may have. More information is contained in the following sections.

What medical information should I receive?

Discharge summary

The hospital will write a discharge summary. This contains all the relevant information about what happened to you and your treatment and recovery in hospital. It will also list the medications you need to take at home. The discharge summary will be sent to your GP and you should be given a copy. If you were already being seen by specialists before your dissection, such as a cardiologist or a vascular consultant, they should also receive a copy of the discharge summary. Make sure the hospital is aware that they should be told.

If you have any unanswered questions (perhaps see your notes on pages 92-95), ask to have them answered before you are discharged from hospital.

Follow-up appointments

Aortic dissection is a serious illness requiring life-long follow-up. Before leaving hospital, ask your medical team who will be responsible for your follow-up. In most cases, you will be asked initially to come back and see the consultant who looked after you in hospital. In the longer term, you may be handed over to another specialist, such as a cardiologist. Make sure that you understand and are happy with your follow-up plan before you leave hospital.

When you are discharged from hospital, or shortly after, you should receive an appointment to see your consultant. This is typically 6-8 weeks after discharge, or three months after an uncomplicated, medically managed Type B dissection. This first appointment is a really important one. Do not miss it. If you cannot attend on the date, call the hospital to make alternative arrangements.

At your follow-up appointment your consultant will review your progress and advise you about the long-term follow-up and monitoring you need.

Further treatment

In some cases, your aortic dissection will require further treatment. For example, if you had surgery, it may not have been possible to repair all of your dissected aorta at once and further surgery may be required. If you had a Type B dissection, sometimes it is better to manage it medically initially, then consider surgery in a few months.

Most patients require life-long surveillance. Your consultant will tell you whether you might need further treatment and what that might be. Regular CT or MRI scans enable the consultant to see your aorta and decide what needs to be done and when.

Any additional surgery would be carefully planned in advance and may be by open surgery or by endovascular treatment using a stent.

Discharge medication and repeat prescriptions

As you leave hospital, you should be given a supply of the medicines you will need to take at home. Your medical team should explain what these medications are and do, when to take them and any side effects to look out for. There is also information within Part B of this Patient Guide. If you have any questions about medication, a pharmacist (at the hospital, GP surgery, or local pharmacy) can help.

Your discharge summary contains the list of the medications that your GP should continue to prescribe for you. When you get home, make an appointment with your GP to arrange for your repeat prescriptions. Ensure you discuss any concerns you have and make a plan with them for your long-term care. As an aortic dissection patient, you may need to see the GP more frequently than you used to.

Pain relief

Good pain control is essential for a speedy recovery and to help you return to normal activities. When you leave hospital you may be given tablets for pain relief. Take them at regular intervals as prescribed and before pain can build up – this is the key to successful pain control. The rule is:

Don't wait for the pain.

If you have had surgery, coughing or sneezing may be painful. If this happens, find a cushion or a rolled-up towel and hold it firmly but carefully against your chest. When trying to sleep, you may find it helps to place a pillow where needed to get comfortable. After surgery on your left side for a Type B dissection, a pillow placed under your armpit and down the left side of your body may enable you to lie on that side comfortably without pain.

When you are feeling more comfortable, you can gradually reduce your pain relief medication. Aches and pains in your chest and shoulders may continue for some months after surgery, perhaps longer in the case of very extensive surgery. If there is any change in the nature and location of your pain, contact your GP.

Constipation

Constipation can occur following surgery or due to pain medications. To help prevent or resolve this, eat a well balanced diet, e.g. with additional fruit and fibre and drink plenty of water. Keeping mobile and taking regular walks will also help.

Once you have been at home for a week, if you are still constipated, seek advice from your GP. They may prescribe a laxative if you need it.

Wounds

If you have had open aortic surgery you will have a wound in the middle of the chest at the front, or at the back between the shoulder blades and down around the left side of the rib cage. You may also have a wound in your groin on either side and some patients will also have a wound near the collar bone. If you have had endovascular surgery, typically you will just have a wound in your groin.

The nurses will check and tend to your wounds regularly until you leave hospital. In general they should heal without problems when you are home. You should be given instructions about how to care for your wounds and change the dressings. It is important to report to a nurse at your GP surgery if you experience any redness, pain or leakage from the wound so that this can be treated. It is possible for wounds to get infected and this needs immediate treatment.

You may have stitches or staples in your wounds or where your chest drains were secured. These need to be removed 7-10 days after your operation. If you are discharged before they have been removed, the ward nurse may arrange for them to be removed by a district nurse or a nurse at your GP surgery. However, as letters can be delayed, you might prefer to book an appointment, rather than wait to be contacted.

Advice on bathing and showering with your wounds is given on page 37.

Once scars have formed over your wounds, you should protect them from the sun with a total block sunscreen. Gently rubbing in a cream such as E45 and gently massaging the area can also assist with healing. If your scar becomes thick, bumpy and raised (sometimes known as keloid scars), you may want to talk to your GP about it.

Complications

Not all aortic dissection patients experience complications, but some do. Complications include stroke, spinal cord injury, loss of voice, heart rhythm disturbance, temporary kidney failure, nerve issues and/or wound infection. Such complications can extend your hospital stay.

Once you are home, any complications will be managed by your medical team alongside caring for your aortic dissection. Treatment of any complications will be specific to you and the detail is beyond the scope of this Guide, however, some general advice is given below under 'Long-term recovery' on page 45.

Ask your doctors about any complications you have had before you leave hospital and make sure you know how they will be treated.

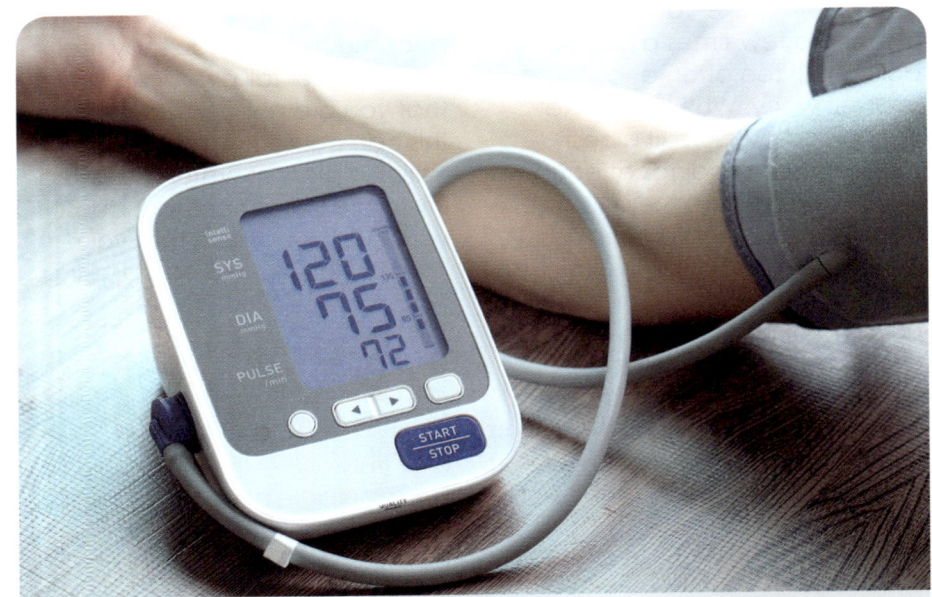

Resting blood pressure and heart rate

An extremely important aspect of your care is to control your blood pressure and heart rate to avoid unnecessary stress on your aorta.

You should monitor your blood pressure and heart rate at home. You can buy a monitor from a pharmacy or online. Choose one that uses an upper arm cuff, not a wrist cuff, and one that is certified for medical use. It is important that you choose one with a cuff that is the correct size for your arm – usually expressed as the circumference of your arm. Cuffs which are too big or too small will not give a correct reading. For further information, the British Heart Foundation produces guidelines on suitable blood pressure monitors – see the Resources section at the end of this Patient Guide.

Typically, the recommendation after an aortic dissection is to aim for a resting blood pressure of 120/80 mmHg and a resting heart rate of 60-70 bpm. If your doctor gives you a different target for your particular case, you should follow that recommendation.

To start with, take your blood pressure a few times a day – but don't do it too often and cause yourself worry. When you take your blood pressure, it is best to take three readings at each session and record the average. To obtain meaningful readings you should rest first for five minutes, be fully relaxed in a sitting position, have no stimulants such as coffee or cigarettes beforehand, keep your legs on the floor and do not cross your legs. Further advice can be found under 'Blood pressure' in the Resources section at the end of this Patient Guide.

Your blood pressure will change depending on the time of day, what you are doing and what medication you have taken. This is completely normal. However, if you are regularly getting readings significantly above your target blood pressure, you should talk to your GP.

To get your blood pressure well-controlled, it may take some months and you may need help from your GP to adjust medications. You may need to be persistent. Once you are confident that your blood pressure is controlled and you are achieving the target figure, you can reduce the amount of self-monitoring that you do. It is best to still check your blood pressure at least once a week.

If your blood pressure or heart rate become too low, you may feel dizzy, faint or fall over. First, check that you are not dehydrated, as this can cause low blood pressure - drink a glass of water if needed. If you are still concerned, consult your GP. It is possible that your medication may need adjusting.

I really didn't know what had happened to me until some time after I was out of hospital and started reading the journal my daughter had kept. I was altogether shocked, amazed, frightened, tearful and grateful to find out I had received a complete new aorta. I had a rough time in hospital and it's been a hard road back to anything like my original fitness and mental state. However, the two words that have kept me going have been hope and determination.

Cliff Grover -
Type A dissection with total repair

Mental and emotional adjustment

After your aortic dissection and discharge from hospital you may have days when you feel low, anxious or irritable.

You may experience nightmares and/or flashbacks (vivid snapshot memories of bad experiences accompanied with feelings of intense anxiety and a sense of 'being back there'), and an increased sense of threat that something bad is going to happen. These are normal responses to trauma and are signs that your brain is trying to process what you have been through and assess whether you are now safe. You may also experience low mood, heightened anxiety and/or irritability, problems sleeping, or other difficulties related to psychological well being.

Try to allow these feelings and experiences to come and go without suppressing them. Remind yourself that you are safe and that these feelings are normal after what you have been through.

If you are concerned about your mental or emotional health, or if these experiences persist longer than 2 to 3 months after discharge, it is important to seek help. Contact your GP for a referral to psychological therapies, which can be extremely effective in alleviating these experiences.

Further information on this subject is available on page 58.

What practical matters should I consider?

Mobility aids

If you have had a long stay in hospital you may still be very weak. Many mobility aids are available. Either the hospital physiotherapist, a community physiotherapist or occupational therapist should assess your needs and, in some cases, will be able to supply you with equipment such as:

- A walking frame or walking stick
- An elevated toilet seat
- Bath rails to help you in and out of the bath
- Support rails
- Special cushions (such as a V-pillow) to help you sleep by avoiding pressure on wounds or ribs
- Stair rails if your stairs do not have adequate rails
- Aids for the kitchen such as jar and tin openers

Most patients need such equipment only temporarily.

Showering or bathing

After surgery, showering or bathing will help to keep your wounds clean and encourage them to heal. Ensure that you rinse off all soap and then pat your wounds dry gently with a clean towel. Do not use a flannel or sponge when cleaning wounds, as these may harbour infection.

When you have a bath or shower, use a non-slip mat. If possible, use a shower rather than a bath for the first few weeks. If you do take a bath, remember:

- Do not add anything to your bath; use water only.
- Empty the water from the bath before you get out, in case you fall.
- Ensure you have a non-slip mat or a towel under you in the bath before attempting to stand up.
- If at all possible, do not get into or out of the bath on your own. Have someone assist you to avoid the risk of slipping or taking too much weight on your arms, which may cause damage.

Rest, sleep and relaxation

During your first few weeks at home, you will find you tire easily. This is completely normal.

Getting plenty of rest is important for your recovery. Take rests during the day. Tell your relatives and friends when your rest periods are so they don't disturb you. If you tire while doing something, such as climbing the stairs, sit down and rest. Notice any self-critical thoughts or negative beliefs about resting as they arise – it is common for some people to push themselves too far during the recovery phase as they find the idea of slowing down and resting extremely challenging. Try and challenge these thoughts by asking yourself what you would say to a friend or loved one if they were recovering from hospital and saying that they should be doing more and shouldn't be resting. It's important to try and show yourself the same compassion you would show a loved one while you move through the recovery process, which will take some time.

Good sleep at night is vital to your recovery. Ideally, try to have at least eight hours of sleep a night. This may be difficult at first because your normal sleeping pattern will have been disturbed while you were in hospital, or you may be in pain and unable to resume your normal sleeping position. It is important to continue taking your pain medication as instructed above to help you sleep.

If you have sleeping problems longer-term, talk to your GP. It may be that emotional trauma or medication are causing sleep difficulties. The NHS websites have excellent advice on sleep.

Diet

The food you eat plays an important part in the healing process. After surgery, it is not unusual for your appetite to be poor in the early weeks. If you cannot face big meals, eat little and often. After three months or so you should be back to your normal eating pattern and have regained much of any weight lost in hospital.

You should always try to follow the principles of healthy eating. For further advice, the hospital may have given you information or a booklet on healthy lifestyle choices. You can also find recommended information in our Resources section at the end of this Patient Guide.

If, in spite of doing these things, you continue to have difficulty with either too much or too little weight, you should consult your GP.

Alcohol

Alcohol may be taken in moderation after discharge from hospital, but you should first ask your nurse or pharmacist for information about alcohol consumption together with your particular medications. In particular, if you are taking warfarin, you should avoid excessive drinking as it will alter your INR (see the section on warfarin on page 72).

If you need or want to reduce your alcohol intake, please discuss this with your nurse before discharge or with your GP.

Smoking

If you were a smoker before your aortic dissection, it is strongly recommended that you give up smoking. If you need help to stop smoking, your GP can tell you how to go about this.

Sexual relations

If you have had an aortic dissection it is common for you and your partner to be anxious about resuming sexual activity. It is quite safe to resume at any time, provided you feel up to it both physically and mentally, and are gentle.

Some men experience problems getting an erection after an aortic dissection. Your GP can help, and you must consult your GP before using medications such as Viagra (sildenafil) as it may not be safe with some of your new medications. It can also affect control of your blood pressure.

Remember there are other ways to be intimate and feel emotionally close to your partner that do not involve penetrative sex and are not affected by aortic dissection. It can be helpful to think of penetrative sex as part of a full range of intimate activities rather than as the 'end goal'.

Flying and holidays

If you need to fly very soon after your dissection, perhaps because you had your dissection abroad, you should obtain a Fit-to-Fly certificate using the forms you can obtain from your airline. Make sure you have several copies each signed by your surgeon or other doctor, in case the airline needs to keep a copy. In some cases the airlines' medical advisers or your travel insurers will have the final say.

You can take a holiday at home in the UK at any time, provided you can cope with the travelling necessary.

For holidays abroad, wait until after the discussion with your consultant at your initial outpatient appointment. You may be advised not to travel abroad, depending on what is happening to your aorta and whether you are likely to need further treatment. Many patients make a full recovery and start off flying short-haul before undertaking long-haul travel.

When sunbathing, cover any scars with total sunblock in the first six months after surgery. Some people find exposing their scar in public very difficult for fear of embarrassment; this is normal and likely to get much easier over time. Remember that other people are rarely looking at us or thinking the things we think they are when we're feeling a little socially anxious. It's a good time to notice the thoughts and feelings that are coming up related to your scar and see if you can gently challenge your thoughts if they're all negative, perhaps reminding yourself that the scar is a sign of survival and resilience.

It is important to provide details of your aortic dissection and any surgery to your travel insurance company to ensure you have adequate health insurance cover abroad. You may need to use an insurer that specialises in cover for people with medical conditions.

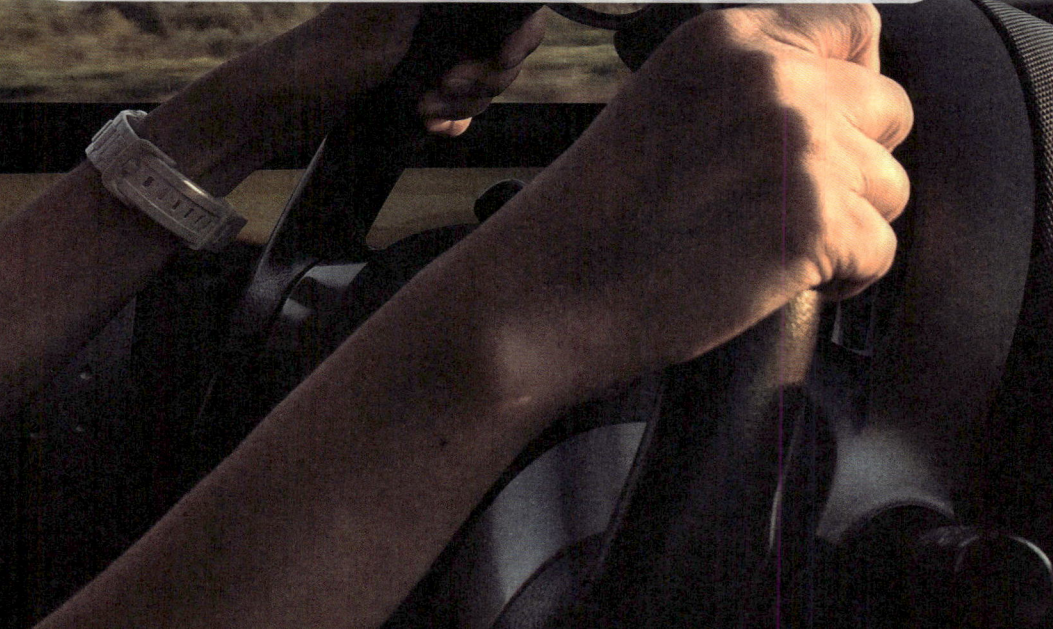

Driving

Ask your medical team for advice about when you can resume driving. If you have had surgery, it is essential that you do not drive until you are sufficiently healed that you can be in full control of a vehicle and can safely perform an emergency stop. Typically, this will be 4-6 weeks after your surgery.

The DVLA has rules for people affected by certain medical conditions. These are stricter for professional drivers. You can be fined for not reporting a medical condition.

Full information is available at the DVLA website: www.gov.uk/health-conditions-and-driving

You also need to notify your insurers that you have had an aortic dissection.

Whether as a driver or as a passenger in a vehicle, you are not exempt from wearing a seat belt. After surgery, you may find it more comfortable to place a folded towel between the seatbelt and your chest.

How should I resume activity at home?

Especially after surgery, most people find that it takes at least 2-3 months to make an initial recovery so that they are able to walk around their home, climb stairs reasonably easily, do short walks outside and help with small household jobs and cooking. This may be quicker, for example, after a Type B dissection which is medically managed, but it may also be longer, depending on the nature and extent of your dissection, surgery and complications.

What about Exercise?

Gentle exercise is an important factor in your initial recovery. This section covers some key aspects.

Patients vary widely in their initial physical capabilities, depending on the type and extent of their dissection or surgery, whether they experienced complications and what medicines they are on. The longer you have spent in hospital, in particular in ICU, the harder exercise will feel to start with. Try to work out with the hospital staff such as the physiotherapist, or with your GP, a suitable exercise regime for you to adopt and anything that you should specifically avoid. Some hospitals have specific rehabilitation teams that you may be able to access.

You may feel shocked and frustrated at how little you can do initially after an aortic dissection. While your progress may seem very slow, in time you will recover many of the capabilities you have lost. Initially, even walking around the house or climbing stairs may be difficult. The first exercise you should take up is walking, starting with short distances, at a slow pace. You can then gradually build up your distance and speed as your recovery progresses.

It is also important to maintain the range of movement in your shoulders, arms and legs, particularly following surgery. You should continue any arm and leg exercises you were shown in the hospital for at least the first month after discharge.

If you experienced breathing problems, you should have been shown deep breathing exercises in hospital. Ensure you keep these up, as it is important to get your full lung function back.

When you feel ready, you can add in small jobs around the house such as preparing meals, and later, slightly more strenuous exercise such as light gardening. Always build up progressively in small steps, avoid lifting or bending too much and ensure you get sufficient rest.

Tiredness and breathlessness when you start exercising are a normal part of the rehabilitation process, as long as it is not distressing for you. A good way to know you are not overdoing things is to ensure that you can talk easily at the same time as exercising.

If you notice yourself becoming easily tired you are probably overdoing things, in which case reduce the extent of your activities. You should also stop doing exercise before you get tired, especially in the early days and weeks after discharge. Always ensure that you rest between periods of exercise and try to get a good night's sleep.

For more information about exercise, including what to do if you need to regain lost strength, refer to the exercise section under 'Long-term recovery' on page 45.

Summary of Part A

You have experienced a serious medical emergency.

Recovering from it will take time, patience and support. There is a lot for you to learn and to do. Try not to feel overwhelmed by it all.

Many patients have been here before you and have shared their knowledge in this Guide to help you. Your job now is to manage yourself and your care the best that you can, so that you make a good recovery.

Start with what you have read in this part A of The Guide and move on to part B when you feel completely ready to do so.

Part B -

Back Home:
Life After
Aortic Dissection

- Long-Term Recovery
- Medications

Long-Term Recovery

How long does recovery take?

Recovery from an aortic dissection can take from a few months up to many years and depends on a number of factors. These include your age, fitness and general health before dissection; the type, location, extent and severity of your dissection; whether you have an underlying genetic condition or other illnesses; whether your dissection requires further intervention; the medications you take; plus your lifestyle, exercise, sleep and food. Your aim should be to return to enjoying a good quality of life, in time.

A good quality of life after aortic dissection may not be the same as the quality of life you enjoyed before aortic dissection. This part of the Patient Guide will help you obtain the best quality of life.

You should remember this:

Quality of life is not a luxury, it is essential. Seek help and do not suffer in silence.

In the first instance, refer to this Guide, along with seeing your doctors for the necessary follow-up consultations. If your quality of life is not what you would like it to be, discuss this with your doctors. They can only help you if they know.

> "Our lives have changed, but life goes on. It can still be full and rewarding, just different. Do not dwell on what you could do but concentrate now on making the most of what you can do. Enjoy life."
>
> *Keith & Lynne Watson*

Who is responsible for my medical care?

Continued care for your dissection, recovery and follow-up is the responsibility of your hospital consultant, who will usually be a cardiac or vascular surgeon, or a cardiologist. This should remain the case for the long term, unless the consultant discharges you from their care back to your GP. Aortic disease must be treated as a condition requiring life-long monitoring; the only exception to this is if there is very good evidence that you are fully recovered and are unlikely to develop any further problems with your aorta. Contact with your consultant will normally be via scheduled follow-up appointments, initially every six months and later, annually.

Apart from this specialist care for your aorta from your hospital consultant, and in an emergency (see below), your GP is responsible for caring for your overall health and should be your first point of contact for any concerns you have.

Your GP can manage your medication, deal with concerns over ongoing or new pain, help with your mental and emotional health and advise you about your recovery generally. If your GP thinks that you should be referred back to your consultant or other services, they will arrange that.

In the first few weeks after you return home, your GP will be guided by the discharge summary from the hospital, which will have been sent to them. As mentioned before, as soon as you feel able, you should make an appointment to see your GP to review your discharge summary, the medications you are on, your care plan and any concerns that you have.

- **In an emergency**, do not hesitate to call 999 for an ambulance or have someone take you immediately to A&E. Tell the ambulance crew and the A&E staff that you have a history of aortic dissection.

- **For non-emergency but urgent problems out-of-hours** ring NHS 111 in England and Wales, NHS 24 on 111 in Scotland. For out-of-hours non-emergency cover in Ireland and Northern Ireland, provision varies by area. You can call your GP's number and listen to the recorded message which should tell you who to call, or preferably find out who to call before any urgent problem might occur.

What monitoring and follow-up can I expect?

In the first year after your aortic dissection, you will probably have one or more CT or MRI scans to check your whole aorta. You may also visit a cardiologist and have an echocardiogram to look at your heart, its valves and the first part of your aorta. You will usually also have a blood pressure check, and an ECG to check your heart rhythm. In subsequent years, it is normal to have these tests annually - aortic dissection is considered to be a condition that requires life-long monitoring. They are very important to check that everything is OK with your aorta. You should not miss your routine scans and appointments.

- **CT scans** – a CT scan gives your doctors a 3D picture of your body. It is like having lots of X-rays all at once. A 'CT aorta' covers the whole aorta from your chest down to your groin and shows your aorta in great detail. CT scans are used to diagnose aortic dissection and to plan aortic surgery, so you may already have had one or more CT scans in hospital. When you have a CT scan, often a substance known as 'contrast' is injected into your arm while you are in the scanner. This enables your doctors to see the structure of your aorta in even greater detail.

- **MRI scans** – an MRI scan is an alternative to a CT scan. It also shows your aorta in great detail, using a different technology that does not involve X-ray radiation. An MRI scan takes longer than a CT scan and is quite noisy. MRI is not yet widely available in all hospitals (and usually not at all in emergency situations). You may be unable to have an MRI scan if you have certain metals within your body, such as a pacemaker.

- **Echo scans** – an echo scan (echocardiogram) uses ultrasound to see your heart, its structures, measurements and function. Echocardiography is quick and useful for assessing your heart and valves, including the aortic valve, and your ascending aorta as it leaves the heart. However, it is not a scan of your whole aorta; for that you need a CT or MRI scan.

The results of your scans will be reviewed by the team caring for you and will be explained to you at your appointment or by letter. If you have any questions about the results, you should ask your medical team.

Should I have cardiac rehabilitation?

In the early days and weeks after leaving hospital, you should have been doing basic exercise such as walking. However, you may not yet be ready to return to your previous exercise levels. Attending cardiac rehabilitation classes is recommended and may help you to progress.

If you have had a Type A dissection you may be offered a programme of cardiac rehabilitation, particularly if you have had a replacement aortic valve or another cardiac issue. However, many patients are not automatically offered cardiac rehab and you may need to ask – talk to your consultant or GP and ask if, as an aortic dissection patient, you can be referred for cardiac rehabilitation.

If you have a medically-managed Type B dissection or have had an endovascular (TEVAR or EVAR) procedure, you probably won't be offered cardiac rehabilitation. You should, however, think about how you can help yourself back to full fitness and also consider the online classes mentioned below.

A cardiac rehabilitation programme typically involves attending two sessions a week for eight weeks during which time you will work on your return to fitness under medical supervision. You will gain fitness during the class and learn the basics of warming up before and cooling down after activity. You will find out what your level of activity should be and how to pace yourself as your fitness improves. You may also receive advice on topics such as healthy eating, relaxation and stress reduction to help your recovery.

If you are unable to get a referral to an NHS cardiac rehabilitation class, you can achieve similar results using an online class, such as the one provided by the British Heart Foundation - see the Resources section at the end of this Patient Guide.

What about returning to work?

It is wise to allow yourself time to make an adequate physical and mental recovery before returning to work. At your first outpatient appointment with your consultant you can discuss the timing of your return to work. This will depend on the type and extent of dissection you had, your rate of recovery and the type of work that you do. If your job is not too physically or mentally demanding, you may be able to return to work within a few weeks or months of your aortic dissection. However, some patients, typically those who have had surgery, can take considerably longer to return to work. Some find that they are unable to work at all. Listen to your body and talk to your GP. You will probably have a good sense of whether or not you feel able to return to the job you were doing.

If you plan to return to work, you should discuss with your employer any ways in which they can make the transition easier. Options include a phased return to work where you start with a few hours or days each week and gradually build up, permanently working reduced hours, changes to your role to limit certain activities, or physical aids and assistance if you require them. Your employer is required by law to take your health into account and make reasonable adjustments to enable you to return to work. Discuss this with your manager, your HR department and your GP when you feel ready. If you experience any difficulties, seek independent advice from an organisation such as Citizens Advice.

"

67 years old, four days in an induced coma following a type A dissection and various complications. Six months later I am walking six miles and swimming 40 lengths. Two years later, no boundaries, life may be not quite perfect but it's not far off. "

Richard Westray

49

What does my future look like?

After an aortic dissection, you and your family may have questions and concerns about your future. It is normal to wonder about questions such as: 'Will this happen again?', 'Might I need further treatment?' and 'How will this affect the length and quality of my life?'.

The answers to these questions will be different, depending on your individual situation. Factors such as the type and extent of your dissection, your age, prior fitness and other medical or genetic factors will all play a part.

The best people to ask are your medical team, particularly your cardiothoracic or vascular surgeons and your immediate post-dissection care team, because they know your individual situation. Some hospitals have a specialist aortic nurse or similar who will be able to specifically deal with these concerns.

After the initial acute phase (in hospital), your degree of recovery will influence the longer-term outcome. You can talk to your GP about this, but some questions may require a referral back to your hospital medical team. Your regular (often annual) review where you discuss the results of your routine CT/MRI scan is a good place to ask these questions.

Many of our members share and discuss their stories in our AD Buddies Facebook group (see the Resources pages at the end of this Guide). You may find it helpful to connect with an AD Buddy similar to you (similar age, dissection type, surgery) who is a little further along the recovery journey. You can compare notes and they can help you know what questions to ask, when to ask them and can give you some idea of the kind of answers you might expect.

Your medical team and Aortic Dissection Awareness UK and Ireland, your patient association, are here to help you with these questions. You will worry less about them if you are properly informed, so the first thing you need to do is find out the facts.

How can I best manage any complications?

Not everyone will experience complications, but the following experiences are common among aortic dissection patients.

Pain

General instructions on pain relief are given in the previous section, and you can continue to follow these as your recovery progresses.

Pain from your dissection should subside with time. Pain from an operation where your chest was opened at the front should subside within 2-3 months. If you had surgery where the surgeon operated through your rib cage at the side, pain may continue for a longer period – pain in the left side and shoulder are common.

In all cases, the principles of pain relief are the same. Take your pain relief medication regularly to stay out of pain, not just when you are in pain and feel you need it. If you want to reduce the amount of pain medication you are taking, do so very slowly over many days or weeks.

If your pain increases at any point, or if you feel it is not improving with time, consult your GP.

Stroke

Some people suffer a stroke, either when their dissection occurs or during or after surgery. A stroke is when a small blood clot or some of the deposit within a blood vessel breaks off and travels towards the brain, blocking the oxygen-rich blood supply that part of the brain needs in order to function. Depending on which part of the brain is affected, this can cause difficulty in speaking, moving or balancing. It is important to receive the right care and rehabilitation for a stroke early in your recovery. Make sure you discuss your particular concerns and needs with your hospital medical team and/or GP.

If you have had a stroke, you should be referred to a stroke clinic, either via the hospital or associated with your GP practice. With professional help, most strokes will resolve to a greater or lesser extent, given time.

The stroke clinic may prescribe exercises to help you recover. You may also be given medications to help resolve the stroke and to minimise the risk of another one happening. These may include anticoagulants and a statin (for further information see page 64 on Medications). You can also help yourself by ensuring that you sleep well, as good sleep has been shown to be crucial in allowing the brain to recover its abilities.

If you continue to experience difficulties, talk to your stroke clinic nurse or your GP.

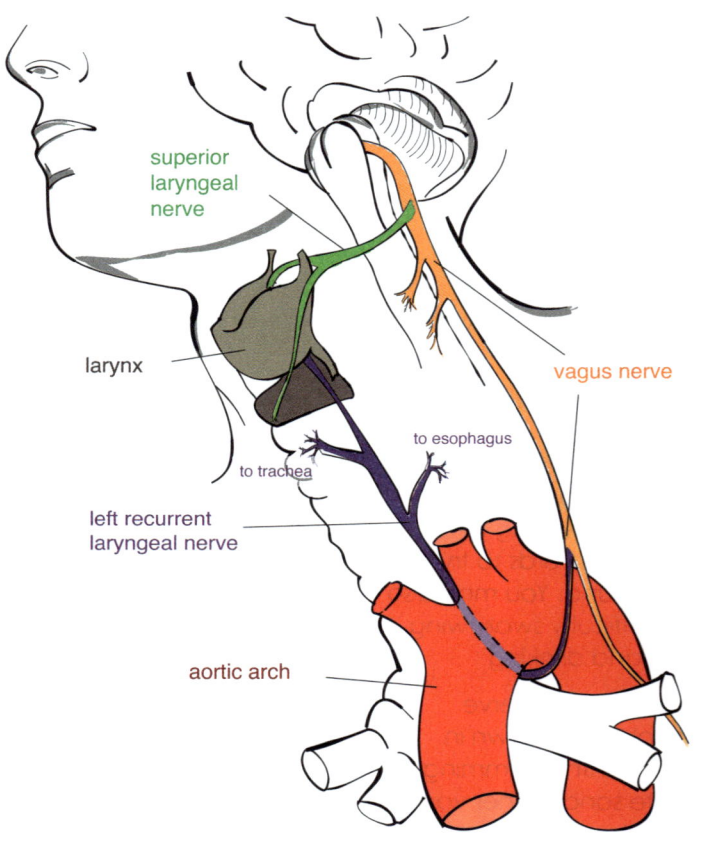

Route of the Left Recurrent Laryngeal Nerve (purple) and its proximity to the aorta

superior laryngeal nerve

larynx

vagus nerve

to esophagus

to trachea

left recurrent laryngeal nerve

aortic arch

Voice and throat

Particularly if you had surgery you may experience difficulty speaking, or the quality of your voice may not be what it was before. There are two main causes of this.

During surgery, you probably had a tube down your throat to help you breathe. This is known as 'intubation'. You may remember this tube coming out, or you may

not. Voice complications are not uncommon after intubation, especially for long periods. They can include sore throat, hoarseness of voice and difficulty swallowing. These are usually minor complications and resolve with time, typically 3-6 months.

If your dissection involved the aortic arch and/or you had extensive open chest surgery, one of the nerves that controls your vocal cords may have been affected. The nerve that controls your left vocal cord loops under the aortic arch and has to be carefully identified and sometimes moved by your surgeon when they repair your aorta. This nerve is called the Left Recurrent Laryngeal Nerve (LRLN) (see diagram opposite).

If this nerve is bruised or injured it can prevent the left vocal cord from closing correctly. You may find that you are hoarse, unable to speak in anything but a whisper or you may find it very tiring forcing air over the vocal cords to try and make a sound. You may also experience difficulty swallowing while eating and drinking.

In most cases, such a nerve injury will resolve on its own in typically 3-6 months. Humming your favourite songs, other vocal exercises, and speech therapy can help. In some cases, it is necessary after six months to see an Ear, Nose & Throat specialist to see if your vocal cords have started to move correctly. If not, you might have a small surgical procedure to reposition the vocal cord and restore your voice. Your GP can make the necessary referrals.

* They are not generally available as NHS classes. Sometimes called 'Phase 4' classes

What exercise can I do long term?

This section contains general advice as to what exercise you can and can't do. In some cases the advice may vary if your medical team has advised you to avoid certain activities.

Once you have started your journey back to fitness by exercising at home after discharge, and have perhaps completed a cardiac rehabilitation class or an online class, you should continue to exercise to gain fitness and strength. This will help with your recovery and enable you to return to as normal a life as possible.

However, whatever exercise you do, it is crucial to work at a pace that suits you and avoid overdoing things. That will often set you back.

Your next stage of exercise can either be by yourself or you can consider joining a community cardiac rehabilitation class. These are typically locally-organised accredited classes(*) and may charge a small fee. They follow a similar pattern to NHS cardiac rehabilitation classes but with an increased level of exercise and more self-supervision. To check if there is such a class in your area, see the Resources section at the end of this Patient Guide.

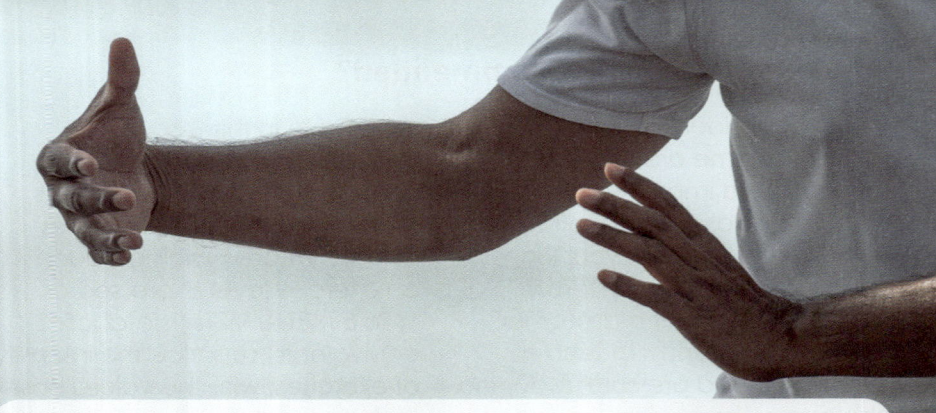

Are there exercises I should not do?

Generally, the advice following an aortic dissection is that you should not lift too much weight.

It is hard to be more specific about what a 'heavy' weight might be after an aortic dissection. This will vary greatly between people depending on the extent of their dissection, their prior fitness, their age and progress in recovery. As a guideline, if lifting causes you to grunt, strain, or jar yourself, then the object is too heavy. Generally, avoid lifting things such as heavy shopping, suitcases or young children.

Whenever you do lift something, ensure you lift correctly, that is, with a straight back and lifting using your legs. Limit yourself to your own easily manageable weight, and avoid straining. Whatever your own situation is, always be mindful of the need not to lift too much and ask for help if in doubt.

Do not take part in 'weight lifting' as a sport.

Do not take part in contact sports such as rugby, football, basketball, or martial arts (*). One reason for this is that you need to avoid raising your blood pressure excessively. In particular, the stress and contact of competitive sports (and 'isometric' exercise such as weight lifting) can cause this. Some sports also involve heavy bodily contact, which is inadvisable as it will jar the body and its internal organs.

Activities such as swimming and tennis which use the upper body a lot are permitted, but you should build up to them slowly.

* Tai Chi is allowable

What exercises are recommended?

The key considerations for your exercise regime are to focus on continued improvement in your cardiovascular condition to benefit your heart, your lungs and your circulatory system. This will also benefit many other aspects of your health such as reducing blood pressure, reducing cholesterol, improving your sleep, and improving recovery after any stress.

Recommended forms of exercise include walking, swimming, cycling, and if and when your recovery permits, more strenuous activities such as gentle running and hill walking. If you previously enjoyed competitive football or basketball, there are walking football and walking basketball clubs which you may like to try.

Further recommendations for acceptable exercise are referred to in the resources listed at the end of this Guide, under 'Exercise'. These sources recommend suitable activities as being those which produce an exercise level expressed as '3 to 5 METs'. METs (metabolic equivalents) describe the intensity of exercises, with the values based on how much each activity increases blood pressure, where a MET of 1 equals resting.

Increase the amount and degree of exercise you do slowly, staying within your capacity as that develops. If you tire yourself out, you will need extra rest and sleep, and you may be surprised by how much. When this happens, there is a natural tendency to try and 'catch up' with missed exercise by doing more exercise, which tires you out even more. This can lead to the 'overactivity/rest cycle' shown in the graph below.

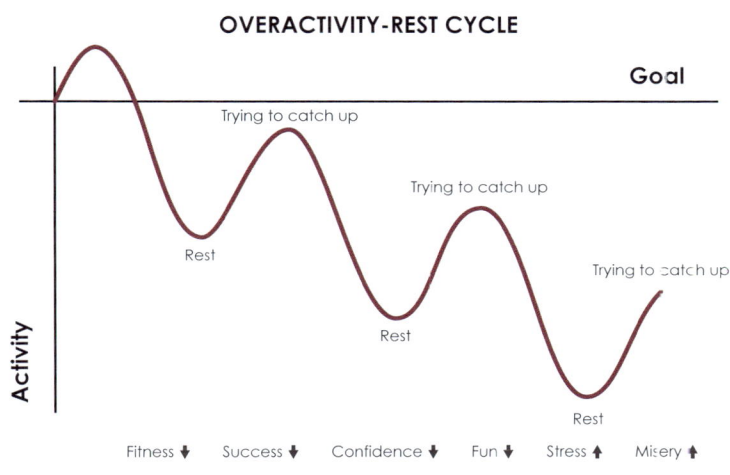

OVERACTIVITY-REST CYCLE

Goal

Trying to catch up

Trying to catch up

Trying to catch up

Rest

Rest

Rest

Activity

Fitness ↓   Success ↓   Confidence ↓   Fun ↓   Stress ↑   Misery ↑

Weeks ➜

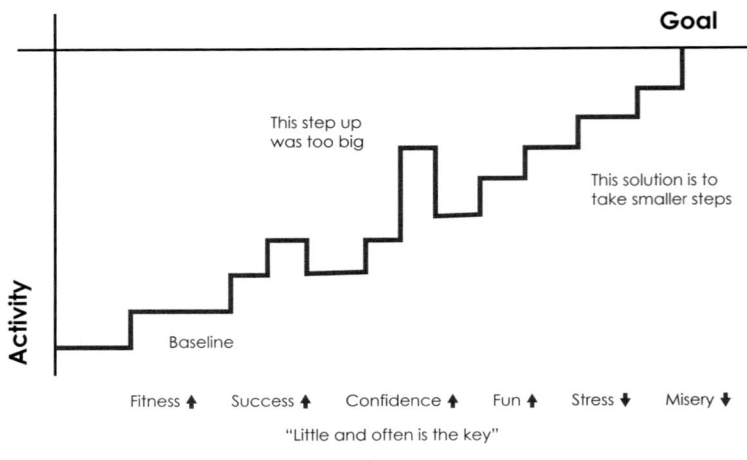

PACING

Goal

This step up
was too big

This solution is to
take smaller steps

Activity

Baseline

Fitness ↑   Success ↑   Confidence ↑   Fun ↑   Stress ↓   Misery ↓

"Little and often is the key"

Weeks ➜

Avoid this by exercising regularly and increasing the intensity in small manageable steps. This is called 'pacing' and is shown in the graph above.

You may be given information about these principles during your cardiac rehabilitation.

You should work up to a recommended amount of exercise of 30 minutes of aerobic exercise for five days a week, totalling 150 minutes a week. You may not be able to achieve this in the early days, even after a cardiac rehabilitation class. However, by following the principles above of pacing and avoiding the overactivity/rest cycle, you should be able to build up to that in time. Once you are comfortably able to achieve 150

minutes per week, you can go on to more exercise if you wish, but you should try and maintain a minimum of 150 minutes per week over the long term.

Try to maintain a regular exercise regime, even if you have to cut back a little on the exertion each time. This is because if you stop exercising for more than a few days you may find your progress has slipped back and you will need to spend time recovering to where you had got to.

Your blood pressure will rise moderately during exercise. This is normal and acceptable. If you are concerned, monitor your blood pressure during and after exercise to check that it is not excessive and that it returns to normal soon after exercise.

How can I regain my lost strength?

If you have lost strength due to your dissection and a long stay in hospital, you should incorporate some gentle muscle-building activities in your exercise, involving your entire body and all sets of muscles. Building muscle in all muscle groups also helps with controlling cholesterol. However, as with all exercise, you must avoid overdoing it.

You must avoid strenuous weight lifting, including bench presses, chest presses, dead lifting or full press-ups, and avoid holding your breath at any time.

Instead, you can do light weight training. You can do this with a range of light exercise weights such as dumbbells, which can be bought at a reasonable cost. You could also use a home gym, or a gym at a public health centre, but again, only use light weights.

You can also do strength training exercises using just your body weight, such as doing sit-to-stand exercises with a chair, or even squats. You can do 'press-ups' initially against a wall, and later, press-ups from your knees. You may have been introduced to many of these options at a cardiac rehabilitation class.

Pilates is also a great way of increasing your 'core strength' and also encourages good breathing practice when lifting etc.

When doing strength training there are two important factors.

Firstly, you should use only light weights and focus on the number of repetitions. Judge what a 'light' weight is by how easy it is to lift at the end of a session. Start with a single set of no more than 10 repetitions (reps), then add in more sets as you are able. You might for example progress to a typical workout of three sets of 10 repetitions of an exercise. As you do this, you should always ensure that the weight you use (or your body-weight exercise selected) is light enough so that the last repetition of the last set remains well within your muscle capacity and nowhere near 'failure'. Similarly, if you find 3 x 10 reps getting easy, you could first increase it to 3 x 15, rather than increasing the weight.

Secondly, ensure you continue to breathe properly when exercising. The best pattern is to breathe in when lowering the weight, then breathe out a long breath as you exert to lift the weight. Never hold your breath.

More information can be found in the Resources section at the back of this Patient Guide, particularly the article 'Recommendations for Exercise for post-Aortic Dissection Patients'.

How should I manage my mental health?

Your mental health is very likely to be affected by the trauma of your aortic dissection and hospital stay. Most people experience a higher degree of anxiety and worry than normal - more than just your concerns about your physical and medical challenges.

The most common experiences are anxiety (about something bad happening again or about future healthcare procedures), worry, depression, shock, trauma, Post Traumatic Stress Disorder (PTSD), sleep problems, a sense of 'why me?', a lack of mental agility, memory issues, and 'post-perfusion syndrome' (sometimes called 'pump-head', which we will come to later in the Guide).

You can achieve a great deal with self-help methods of managing your mental health, and there are some tips here. However, many people get professional help, and it is important to do so if you are struggling, as trained counsellors and therapists are familiar with the issues you may experience and can help you through them. Your GP can refer you, but you do need to tell them.

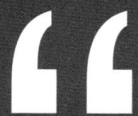

I was 46 when I had my Type A aortic dissection in October 2018. One minute I was sitting down for a meeting and the next I was waking up in a hospital bed and being told that it was four days later, and I had had life-saving open-heart surgery for a condition I hadn't even heard of! My journey away from that day and towards the 'new me' has been a long and, at times, painful one but I hope that as long as I keep taking my blood pressure medication every day and having my annual CT scans, this new me will have a long and fruitful life.

Alex Williams

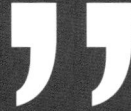

The main mental and emotional effects you may experience are:

Trauma-related difficulties

It is normal to experience some trauma-related difficulties following discharge from hospital, for example related to the experience of the aortic dissection and/or experiences in ICU. Most patients experience a degree of anxiety and shock, simply due to the nature of aortic dissections and medical interventions needed. This is sometimes called Post-Traumatic Stress (PTS). Over time, with love, support, and space to process what happened with self-compassion, your traumatic memories and feelings are likely to eventually reduce.

About 30% of aortic dissection patients experience the more serious condition of Post Traumatic Stress Disorder (PTSD). PTSD is characterised by a number of symptoms, which if they 'cluster' together give an even stronger indication of the condition. These are:

1. Re-experiencing – the key indicator of PTSD is if you re-experience the traumatic events which happened to you. This is often in the form of nightmares or flashbacks that include a sense of 'being back there', i.e that the trauma is happening now and there is a feeling of current threat and danger with an intense fear;

2. Avoidance and numbing – the avoidance of trauma reminders and the numbing of emotions;

3. Hyperarousal – anxiety, difficulty concentrating, irritability, and 'hypervigilance' to threat.

It is important to differentiate between trauma-related stress (PTS) and PTSD. Not every case of trauma will lead to PTSD. If you are concerned you have developed PTSD, speak to your GP or your hospital team to assess whether it is appropriate for you to be referred to an NHS Psychological Therapies Service.

The NICE (National Institute for Health and Care Excellence) recommended psychological therapies for PTSD are Trauma-Focused Cognitive Behavioural Therapy, Eye Movement Desensitisation Reprocessing (EMDR) and Narrative Exposure Therapy (NET) – for more information see the Resources section at the end of this Patient Guide.

An excellent introduction to CBT for PTSD is provided by the Psychology Tools website (see the Resources section). The booklet they publish includes a short self-test to give you a better idea of whether your condition is PTSD or not. The booklet also covers some of the basics of the methods used. The strategies mentioned in the booklet include 'grounding' strategies to cope with re-experiencing and finding ways to still do the things that matter to you while you manage symptoms of PTSD. These strategies can be extremely helpful, especially if there is a significant wait to be seen by local NHS services.

Non-NHS services are also available and you should ensure anyone you see is properly qualified.

Anxiety and depression

Anxiety and depression are also common in aortic dissection patients. If you are affected by these and are struggling to manage, do not suffer in silence – seek professional guidance and treatment. You can ask your GP or hospital team for a referral for assessment by a professional psychologist. There is a good evidence base for psychological therapies helping with anxiety and low mood; some people benefit from combining antidepressant or anti-anxiety medication with psychological therapies.

Emotional self-help

If you are reading this Guide, you will realise that you are not alone on your aortic dissection journey. Many other people are on the same journey and would love to talk with you and help you. You can find these people at the national patient association, Aortic Dissection Awareness UK & Ireland, which is run by patients, for patients like you.

Contact us, and benefit from being put in touch with others who have been through similar events. See the Resources section at the end of this Patient Guide.

Two techniques from CBT can really help reduce your anxiety and stress. They are progressive muscle relaxation and relaxed breathing. The Resources section has a link to the Psychology Tools website page on progressive muscle relaxation and relaxed breathing. You can also download .mp3 recordings of these exercises.

There are also other internet resources and mobile phone apps which can assist you with self-help (see the Resources section).

"

Don't let yesterday use up too much of today.

Simon Jones

"

Part B

What about sleep?

It is normal to experience some problems sleeping during and immediately after a hospital admission, but if these persist into your recovery period, you should try some of the following.

Start with self-help methods such as good sleep practices, sometimes called 'sleep hygiene'. In addition, CBT for insomnia (CBT-i) is a proven method to reduce sleeping problems and courses are available (see the Resources section at the end of this Patient Guide).

If problems sleeping persist, seek professional help via your GP. There may be medical reasons, such as medication or other factors which are making your sleep difficult. Even if there are not, CBT-i works best in conjunction with monitoring and support from a professional therapist.

GPs now rarely prescribe sleeping pills to treat insomnia. Sleeping pills can have serious side effects and you can become dependent on them. Sleeping pills are only prescribed for a few days, or weeks at the most, if your insomnia is very bad and other treatments have not worked.

Mental agility and memory

If you have had open surgery for a Type A dissection, you may have been put on a heart-bypass machine during the operation. This keeps oxygenated blood flowing to your brain and vital organs while your aorta is repaired. Sometimes this can affect your mental agility and memory after your operation, especially if you were 'on bypass' for a long time. It is also possible that when you initially had your dissection, the supply of oxygenated blood to your brain was disrupted.

In these cases, you may notice some subtle effects on your mental agility, memory and ability to concentrate. You might feel a bit slower mentally, and perhaps drop things more often than you used to. These effects are sometimes called 'post-perfusion syndrome' or, colloquially, 'pump-head'. These effects are usually subtle and you may just feel that something is not quite right. The effects typically settle down in time. Mental and physical exercise, sleeping well, and healthy eating are all important in recovering your abilities. If you remain concerned about any aspect of your mental health, always see your GP.

What about dental work?

If you have had your aortic valve replaced (with a mechanical or tissue valve) it is important to prevent infection in the valve. This can happen if bacteria are introduced directly into the bloodstream, but it is normally a very low risk. To protect against infection, the most important thing is that you get into the habit of practising good dental hygiene. This means flossing or using interdental brushes twice a day, as well as brushing and seeing the dental hygienist every six months as well as the dentist.

You may also need to take a single antibiotic dose one hour before having any dental work done, including cleaning. Antibiotics are not necessary for just a check-up. Your dentist will provide you with the necessary information and a prescription for the necessary antibiotics when required. More information on this, including the relevant NICE Guidelines, can be found in the Resources section at the end of this Patient Guide.

In addition to an artificial valve, there are certain other rare situations where your hospital consultant may advise you to take precautions against infection; they will inform you of this.

Medications

How should I best manage my medications long-term?

Medications can help you recover from your aortic dissection, manage any residual dissection(*) , help with your day-to-day living and quality of life and protect you from harm in the long term. You will probably need to take a combination of different medications. Some of these will be for life. This section summarises what you need to know.

Taking the right medication properly can help to:

- Keep your blood pressure and heart rate under control
- Reduce the stress and load on your aorta
- Help to 'thin' your blood if required, such as if you received a mechanical aortic valve, or you had an arrhythmia or a stroke
- Remove fluid build-up in your lungs, your chest, or your legs
- Keep you free from pain
- Prevent your condition from getting worse
- Improve your life expectancy
- Improve your quality of life.

Once out of hospital, your GP will be your first point of contact about medications and will work together with your hospital consultant(s) as needed. Your doctors will monitor and review your medications from time to time and may change the dose of a medication or give you a different one, depending on your condition and symptoms.

When talking to any medical staff it is important that they know all the medications you are taking, including the name, dose and frequency, and any changes to your prescription. Keep a careful note of your medications and ensure the list is up to date. Keep a record of what medications you have been prescribed and when, so that you can keep track of changes over time and discuss with your doctors if needed.

A residual dissection is a dissection in any part of the aorta that has not been repaired.

What are all my medications for?

The following descriptions are basic explanations of what the common medications for aortic dissection do. For full information, read the patient information leaflet that comes with every medication and speak with your GP or nurse if you have any questions or concerns. You can also consult the NHS website pages on medications.

Will I have side effects from my medications?

All medications can have side effects although not everyone experiences them. Some side effects are extremely rare, others are more common. A lot of side effects are temporary, occurring only as you get used to a new medication and then going away after a short while.

Tell your GP about any side effects that you get, especially when you notice them for the first time. Some side effects can be unpleasant, but the effects of not taking your medication can be worse. Do not stop taking your medication without first consulting your GP. It may be possible for a doctor or nurse to adjust the dosage or change you to a different medication in order to reduce your side effects.

Pain medications

The advice on pain relief once you are out of hospital remains the same as given in the above sections.

The mainstay of pain relief once out of hospital is paracetamol. You should check with your GP about using paracetamol, but it is generally safe and you were probably prescribed paracetamol as a discharge medication. It should be taken regularly and at the full dose.

Again: **don't wait for the pain.**

You should consult your GP about whether you can use aspirin, especially if you are on warfarin or other anticoagulants such as Rivaroxiban.

You should generally not take painkillers of the 'NSAID' type (non-steroidal anti-inflammatory drug), such as Ibuprofen, Naproxen and Diclofenac, due to the effect they may have on your kidneys and blood pressure in the long-term. However, your GP may decide that they are suitable for you under specific circumstances, perhaps used as a gel, for muscle pain.

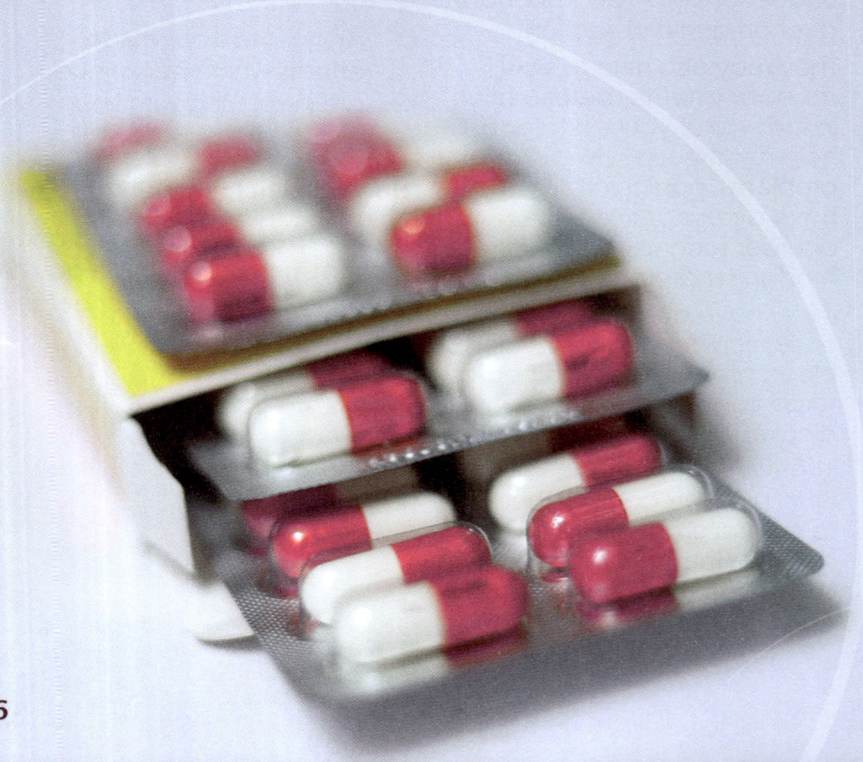

Other medications

The following are the commonest medications after an aortic dissection.

Beta blockers

Examples are: Bisoprolol, Atenolol, Carvedilol, Metoprolol, Nebivolol

What are they for?

Beta blockers help the heart to beat more slowly and less forcefully.

- They reduce the force of your heart's pumping, which helps to reduce the strain on your heart, reduce your blood pressure and heart rate and reduce the stress on your aorta. Keeping your blood pressure and heart rate well under control is very important after an aortic dissection.

- They may also help to slow down any further deterioration in the wall of your aorta and help minimise the risk of future problems, particularly if you have a connective tissue disorder such as Marfan syndrome.

- If you have a residual dissection, the reduction in blood pressure and the heart's force from taking a beta blocker will also help the 'false lumen' to shrink.

- Beta blockers can also help to control problems with your heart rhythm and reduce the discomfort these can cause.

What are the main side effects?

- Tiredness, usually only for the first few days of starting this medication or increasing the dose, but it may persist

- Dizziness or fainting

- Mood swings when you first start taking the beta blockers

- Shortness of breath

- Disturbed sleep

- Cold hands and feet

- If you have asthma, beta blockers may make it worse.

Which side effects should I tell my doctor or nurse about?

- Any of the above side effects which persist and are interfering with your quality of life.

How can I help myself?

If you experience tiredness and lack of energy during the day, try taking your beta blocker before bed to see if that helps.

ACE inhibitors

Examples are: Ramipril, Captopril, Enalapril, Lisinopril, Perindopril

What are they for?

ACE inhibitors have a relaxing effect on the arteries. This lightens the workload of your heart and makes it easier for your heart to pump blood around your body.

After an aortic dissection their main effects are to:

- Lower your blood pressure
- Increase your chances of living longer if your heart muscle function has been affected
- Improve the amount of exercise you can do if your heart muscle function has been affected

What are the main side effects?

ACE inhibitors tend to have very few side effects but the following are possible:

- Irritating cough
- Dizziness
- Impairment in kidney function in susceptible people

If you get any of the following side effects, seek urgent medical attention or call 999:

- Swollen face, lips or mouth
- A severe rash or itching
- Sudden wheezing or problems with breathing

Angiotensin II receptor antagonists (ARBs)*

Examples are: Losartan, Irbesartan, Candesartan, Valsartan

What are they for?

ARBs work in a similar way to ACE inhibitors to lower your blood pressure and provide a protective effect on your aorta, but they are less likely to cause an irritating cough.

What are the main side effects?

Again, ARBs have very few side effects but the following are possible:

- Dizziness
- A decrease in blood pressure

*ARB: 'Angiotensin receptor blockers'

Diuretics

Examples are: Furosemide, Bumetanide, Bendroflumethiazide

What are they for?

Diuretics are sometimes called 'water tablets'. They help your kidneys get rid of excess fluid by making you pass more urine. By doing this, they can also reduce your blood volume and hence reduce your blood pressure. As a result, the heart does not have to work as hard to pump blood around the body. Diuretics can:

- Reduce swelling in your ankles, legs and other parts of your body
- Relieve shortness of breath
- Lower blood pressure
- Help ACE inhibitors and beta blockers to work better.

What are the main side effects?

- Going to the toilet more during the day and possibly at night
- Dizziness or light-headedness
- Dehydration

Which side effects should I tell my doctor or nurse about?

- Any difficulty passing urine
- Passing much less urine than normal
- Constipation
- Pain in your joints
- Dizziness, light-headedness, fainting or blackouts.

How can I help myself?

Try to take your diuretics in the morning and, if you have two doses per day, take them in the morning and in the early afternoon. This will minimise the need to get up to the toilet during the night.

If you have to travel or be somewhere without easy access to a toilet, consider delaying taking your diuretic until later. If you miss or delay taking a dose by more than about three hours, check what the patient information leaflet says about missed doses or check with your GP for what their advice is.

Aldosterone antagonists*

Examples are:
Spironolactone, Eplerenone

What are they for?

These medicines are used to help prevent and treat the build-up of fluid in the body. They work by helping to block the effect of a hormone called aldosterone. They have a mild diuretic effect (which means that they help you to get rid of excess fluid by passing more urine). They are traditionally to help with heart failure but also have beneficial effects after aortic dissection. In particular, they are used in the treatment of difficult-to-control high blood pressure or low blood potassium that does not improve with supplements.

If you are taking ACE inhibitors or beta blockers but your blood pressure is not responding adequately, you may be prescribed one of these medications. It also depends on your symptoms and how severe your condition is.

What are the main side effects?

- Passing less water than usual
- Spironolactone can sometimes cause swelling and tenderness of the breast tissue in men. If this happens, you can be switched to Eplerenone.
- Diarrhoea
- Reduced kidney function
- Dehydration

*Also called mineralocorticoid receptor antagonists, MRAs

Statins

Examples are: Atorvastatin, Simvastatin, Rosuvastatin,

What are they for?

Statins lower the level of cholesterol in your blood and reduce your risk of a heart attack and stroke. In aortic dissection they will also reduce the risk of atherosclerosis build-up inside your aorta, which can cause further problems. If you had a measure of cardiovascular disease before your dissection, using statins for protection is known as 'secondary prevention' and is particularly important after your dissection.

What are the main side effects?

- Muscle aches, cramps and weakness
- Headache
- Nausea
- Diarrhoea

Which side effects should I tell my doctor or nurse about?

- If you have any signs of unusual muscle pain, cramps or weakness, or dark urine, tell your doctor or nurse immediately.

Warfarin

What is it for?

If you have been fitted with a mechanical aortic valve during surgery, the surfaces of the valve must be protected from blood clots forming on them and in the crevices, which would interfere with the working of the valve. Clots can also pass to the brain, causing a stroke. Therefore when you have a mechanical aortic valve, you must take warfarin for life. Other anticoagulants (sometimes called direct oral anticoagulants, or DOACs) are not suitable for this use. Anticoagulants are sometimes known as 'blood thinners'.

Vitamin K in your blood helps it to clot. Warfarin works by interfering with the production of vitamin K.

Warfarin may also be prescribed if you experience atrial fibrillation (AF) after your dissection or surgery, to reduce the risk of a stroke. In this case, you will need to take it until the AF stops and for a short period thereafter. (*)

What tests do I need?

You will need regular blood tests to check how much warfarin you need. These are done at an anticoagulation clinic, either at your GP surgery or at a specific clinic. These checks are needed to ensure your blood remains in an acceptable range for clotting: this is measured by the 'INR', or International Normal Ratio. If your INR is not high enough, your blood will clot too much and risk affecting your valve or causing other problems. If your INR is too high, your blood will not clot enough and may cause excessive bleeding if you cut yourself. Normal blood has an INR of 1.0. For most modern aortic valves, the recommended INR range is 2.0 to 3.0. In some cases, an INR range of 2.5 to 3.5 is recommended.

*If you do not have a mechanical aortic (or other) valve, but you have another reason to need anticoagulation, such as you experience atrial fibrillation, you may be prescribed a Direct Oral Anticoagulant, or DOAC. DOACs also need careful management but require less testing. If you have questions on this, talk to your GP.

It is important to minimise the time that your INR is 'out of range'. It is particularly important not to go below the lower number for long. If this happens, your warfarin clinic should increase your warfarin dose and call you back for a recheck around three days later to ensure that the increased dose is being effective. If your INR is too low for any length of time you may need to have injections of another anticoagulant (heparin) until your INR is back in the recommended range.

What else do I need to know?

You will receive a yellow NHS 'Oral Anticoagulation Therapy' record booklet, in which your blood results will be recorded. Always take your yellow booklet with you to clinic appointments; it has your NHS number in it, plus the history of your INR.

Make sure you tell anyone treating you, such as your GP, your dentist, a pharmacist, or a paramedic, that you're taking warfarin. Some people choose to wear a medic alert bracelet or tag to notify healthcare professionals that they are on warfarin.

Always check before taking any new medication because some medications can affect the way that warfarin works and can change your INR.

Avoid cranberries and cranberry juice, as these foods can increase the anticoagulant effect of warfarin. Also, avoid eating large quantities (especially at irregular intervals) of foods high in vitamin K, such as liver, brussels sprouts, broccoli and dark green vegetables. These can prevent warfarin working as well as it should. This doesn't mean that you should stop eating such foods, but that you should avoid eating large quantities in one go. If you eat a reasonable quantity regularly, the steady effect on your INR will be seen at your regular tests and your warfarin level can be adjusted accordingly.

Alcohol can also affect the level of warfarin in your blood, so it is important to ensure you drink within national recommended guidelines and avoid excessive amounts, particularly binge drinking. Talk to your doctor or nurse for advice.

Home testing

It is possible to test your own INR at home, using a CoaguChek® device. This is done in conjunction with your warfarin clinic. You test your own blood and phone in your INR result, after which you are told of any change in warfarin dosage and when you should next check your blood.

Home testing is of great advantage where access to your clinic is difficult for any reason. It also allows you to continue testing your blood when you go away on a trip or on holiday. Using the home testing device needs training and a supply of testing strips. Ask your warfarin clinic nurse whether they think this would be possible for you.

Further information, including references to the NICE guidelines on home INR testing, can be found in the Resources section at the end of this Patient Guide.

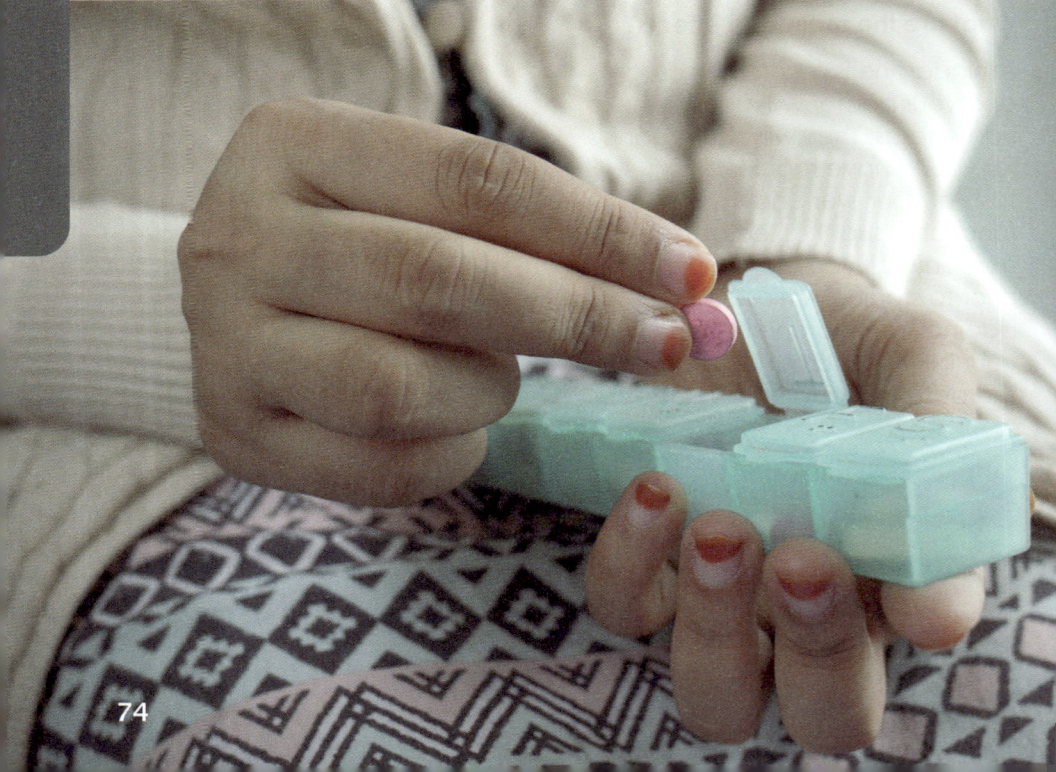

Amiodarone

What is it for?

Amiodarone is an anti-arrhythmic drug used to correct a faulty heart rhythm, including atrial fibrillation (AF). You may experience AF after your dissection or surgery, due to inflammation of the heart. If your AF persists, you will be started on a high dose of Amiodarone for two weeks called a 'loading dose', to get the medication levels in your body up to an effective level for your faulty heart rhythm. After that, your dose will be reduced to a lower level, called the 'maintenance dose'. Subsequent management will be carried out between your cardiologist and your GP.

What are the main side effects?

Amiodarone is a complex drug and your doctor will monitor the side effects. They will also organise for you to have regular blood tests of your liver and thyroid function, usually at least every six months. If you are on warfarin prior to starting Amiodarone, adding Amiodarone may put your INR up and hence reduce the dose of warfarin you need.

What can I do to help myself?

- Stay out of direct sun, especially strong sunlight, and use a high-factor sun block cream if you have to go out in the sun.
- Familiarise yourself with the patient information leaflet and follow it carefully.
- Ensure you get your regular liver and thyroid blood tests.

Part C -
For Family And Carers

- How Can Family, Carers And Friends Help?
- Why Do Families Need Genetic Screening?

How Can Family, Carers And Friends Help?

If a loved one, a friend, or someone you care for has an aortic dissection, it can be a very worrying time and can put a great deal of stress on you. This section covers some of the aspects which can affect you and gives advice on how you can help and understand your loved one's situation, and how to look after yourselves.

What should we expect up to the point of discharge?

How to communicate with the medical team

There will be a lot of questions that you and your family and any carers will want to ask about your aortic dissection and your care.

To ensure communication is as clear and efficient as possible, it is important to nominate one family member to communicate with medical, nursing and ICU staff. This helps to avoid answers being interpreted differently via different routes. It is also difficult for medical staff to have too many people asking the same questions.

It may not be possible for the nominated family member to always speak to the same staff member, perhaps due to shift changes and availability. Nevertheless, having a nominated family member will help to ensure clarity and consistency. Some hospitals are now creating a position of aortic specialist nurse and, where this applies, they will be your medical first point of contact.

If the family is concerned about anything, the nominated family member should speak to either medical or nursing staff straightaway, rather than waiting and worrying. A lot of the waiting for things to happen is unavoidable, but the worrying can be managed.

How to look after yourselves

It is very important for you, as a patient's loved ones, to care for yourselves. It is understandable that you may want to do as much as possible to help your loved one, or be at their bedside at all times.

You might, however, feel very frightened for your loved one or for yourself, or you may find waiting for information from the hospital is physically and mentally exhausting. Many aortic dissections happen to someone who is a parent, hence the dissection also affects the whole family – not just the spouse or partner, but also children and other relatives.

Peoples' responses vary widely to such a life-threatening event for their loved one. Some are very keen to help and support their loved one in hospital, but some people find the events so distressing they can withdraw or not want to know what is happening. Different family members can also react in different ways to the event.

Try to be realistic about how much you can do, and be kind to yourselves. You will probably find it difficult to balance the conflicting wish to support your loved one with all the normal and pressing matters in life, such as work and supporting your family.

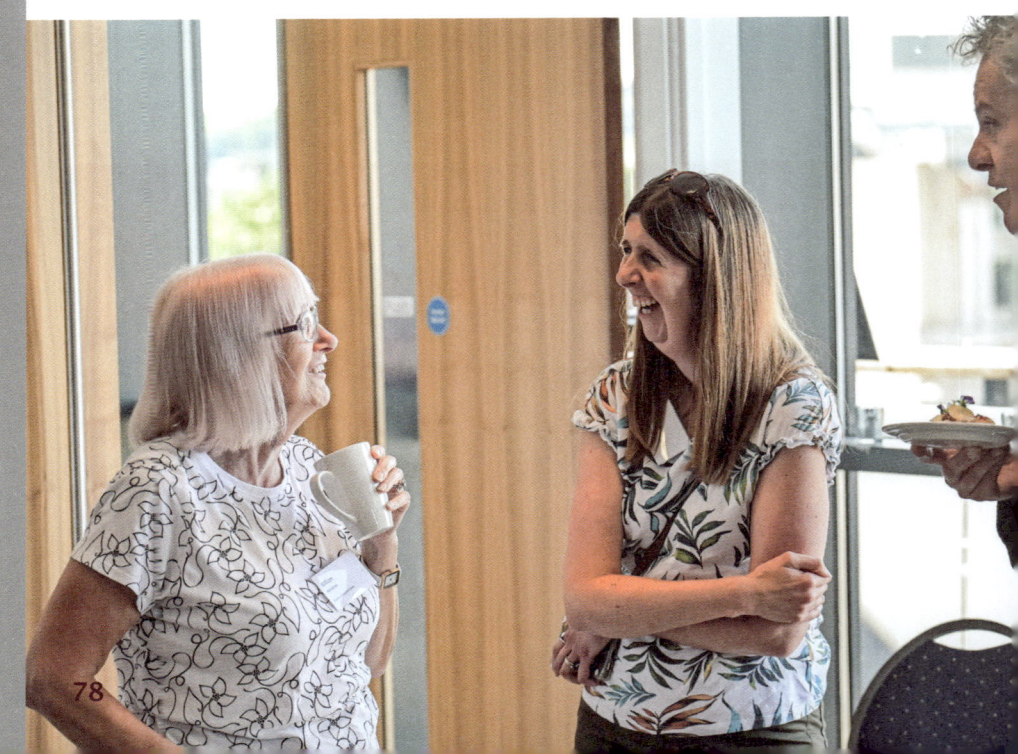

78

Your family member is being cared for by the entire medical team but there are things that you can help with, both for them and for yourself.

Firstly, pace yourself and what you do. Seeing someone through an aortic dissection and afterwards is a long-term effort. Make sure you don't wear yourself out. Take time out for yourself occasionally, to recharge your batteries by doing something you love. This is not selfish or uncaring. It is an essential factor in being able to cope. If you can't cope yourself, you won't be able to help your loved one.

Secondly, don't assume that those around you feel the same as you do. Children may need particular understanding and respect as to the effects on them; some will want to get actively involved, some will not.

Thirdly, when you can, simply be with your loved one who has had a dissection, and help to support them in whatever way is possible. Even if they are not apparently conscious, you can talk with them and perhaps hold their hand. Be cheerful, tell them about your day. But remember they also need sufficient time to rest, sleep, eat and be tended to by the medical staff. Respect the hospital's rules on visiting times and protected meal times, as these are there for a purpose. Don't take offence if the staff ask you to leave for any reason – take that chance to get some rest yourself.

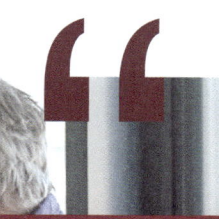

> My husband had a type A dissection in 2005 – it meant emergency open heart surgery and changed our lives forever, but not all for the worse. Thanks to the NHS, he's doing pretty well, and we appreciate the little things in life so much more.
>
> *Rachel & Tim Knight*

What things can we do to help?

You can help by bringing in things to keep your loved one occupied. This might be their smartphone or tablet, to keep in touch with people or to listen to music on earphones. Don't forget the charger and cable. Any food you bring should be checked first with the nursing staff as your loved one may have particular dietary requirements. Do not take in flowers, as most hospitals do not allow them, but your loved one may like to have a family photo or a photo of their pet. It can also help to take in familiar toiletries or a favourite cushion. All these things can help to restore a degree of familiarity and normality.

You can also read the earlier sections of this Guide to help you understand some of what your loved one is experiencing and talk with them about it. They may struggle to take much of it in, initially. Don't force it, take your time and be sensitive to what they want to know first.

Another practical thing you can do is to keep a daily journal or diary. Often, an aortic dissection patient will be completely unaware, or will not remember, much of what has happened, even if they were conscious at the time. This is normal. A journal can be very helpful in helping them make sense of it all. Record what

has been happening day to day, the progress your loved one is making. Maybe include some photos.

This journal can also be useful for your loved one (if they wish) to look back over it in the months after leaving hospital. It can help them understand what happened and adjust mentally. They might want to continue with the journal themselves as their recovery progresses. It can be a source of comfort as recovery progresses, showing progress and providing encouragement for further rehabilitation. However, a journal may not be for everyone.

Finally, stay positive and look forward to normal life returning.

What happens after discharge?

The first few days after returning home will be a learning process for your loved one (the patient), and anyone living with them. It is likely that the burden on the family or carer will increase. Also, the patient will start learning how to manage their condition and to understand their, perhaps slow, rate of progress.

The patient may need physical help with things like bathing, toilet, and going out. They will also need time during the day to rest and sleep. Where the patient remains very weak, they and their family may have to learn to manage things the patient needs, like

80

having a walking frame or stick within reach or needing a toilet booster seat.

Some patients may need help to organise their medications, such as filling pill dispensers correctly, and ensuring repeat prescription requests are submitted and medicines collected.

It is important for both the patient and their loved ones to talk about what their needs are and work out together how to manage the patient's recovery. Things will be different for some time, in many cases, forever. Recognise that you will all need time to recover emotionally from the events surrounding the aortic dissection. It is quite common for people to feel a little low or more emotional than usual once home from hospital – try and allow these feelings to exist and be kind to yourself and each other, reminding yourself that you have been through an ordeal and it will take time to recover physically and psychologically.

Once early arrangements become settled, the patient may need some encouragement to get back to normal. Try not to be over-protective, as this may not be beneficial. For example, it should be perfectly alright for the recovering person to be left alone for some periods during the day, while their family/carers are out (e.g. shopping or working).

The patient should be encouraged and supported in taking appropriate movement or exercise, in finding time and space to get enough rest, eating a balanced diet and, if necessary, giving up smoking. These are all things that supportive family and friends can help and potentially join in with.

The patient and family may receive visits from friends and other relatives. You should make it clear that while you welcome such visits, the patient needs their rest and that you and they will not be able to act as a normal social host might do, such as serving drinks or food. Even sitting and chatting can be extremely tiring for the patient, especially in the early days, so visits may need to be limited.

It can be helpful to involve visitors by letting them know specific things that they can help with, such as a bit of shopping, bringing a meal if you are finding it difficult to cook, doing a bit of cleaning, or that essential piece of maintenance that is needed. Even small practical matters can be a big worry but are easily resolved by supportive friends and family.

> " I remember the ambulance crew saying 'hold on, it's gonna get noisy and bumpy' and the journey back from my dissection was. But with the love of my wife and the fantastic care I received from the NHS staff I made it.
>
> **Stephen Wren** "

Long-term support

The degree of long-term support needed for someone who has had an aortic dissection will depend on the progress they make with rehabilitation. Some will continue to require considerable support while others will return to a more normal life relatively soon. In any case, it is helpful for the patient not to feel that they are dealing with their new life on their own and that they have help and support when needed, physically, practically and emotionally.

Can PTS or PTSD affect my family?

Although the patient is usually thought of as the one at risk of traumatic stress outcomes after an aortic dissection, family members can also be affected. You will naturally be affected if you are caring for someone with PTSD. However, you may experience PTS or PTSD yourself since you have witnessed a traumatic event happen to someone else.

If you, as a family member, are experiencing significant post-traumatic stress yourself, you may also benefit from the resources listed in the Resources section at the end of this Patient Guide, or from a referral to a psychological therapies service or counselling. Talk to your GP about this.

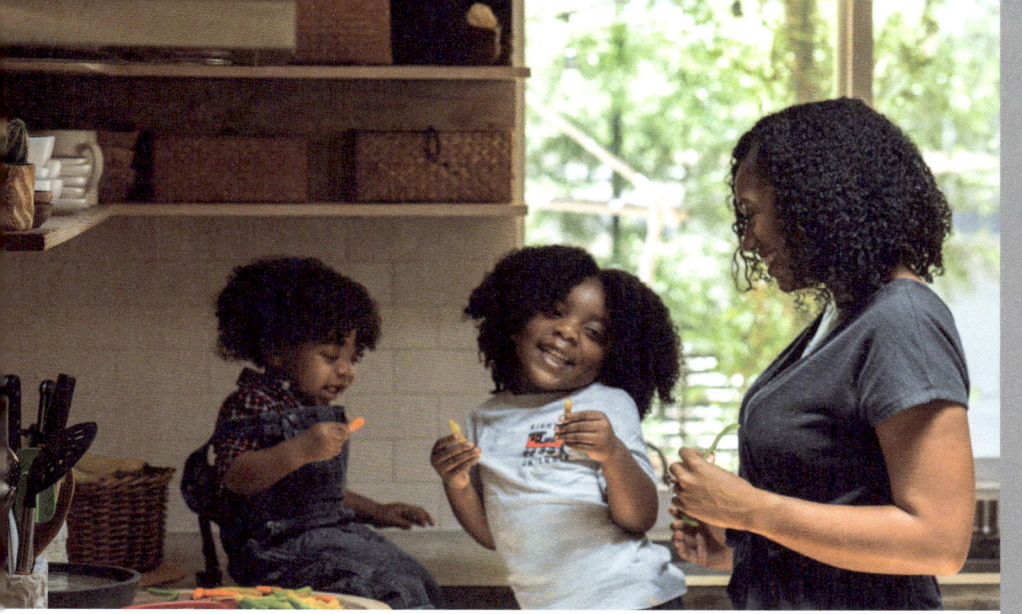

Why Do Families Need Genetic Screening?

As discussed in Part A, some people have a genetic predisposition to aortic dissection and this can therefore run in your family. If you have had a dissection at a relatively young age (typically less than 60 years old), it is particularly important to find out if there are any genetic factors involved and whether any of your relatives may be affected. This is sometimes called genetic 'screening'.

Your hospital team or GP can refer you to an NHS or regional genetics service or inherited cardiac conditions centre. There, experts in genetics will discuss your aortic dissection, take a family history and if necessary, arrange for screening. This may involve genetic testing and imaging (i.e. CT or echo scans) for you and other family members.

"

My father had Marfan syndrome and died of an aortic dissection aged 49, when I was 11. When I had a similar dissection aged 50, it was a very worrying time for my family, including my youngest son, who inherited Marfan syndrome from me. However, due to medical advances in aortic dissection in recent decades, I was able to have life-saving surgery at a specialist centre and a great outcome.

Gareth Owens

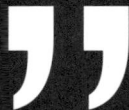

Genetic testing needs careful thought and discussion as it can lead to significant discoveries about you and your family's health. It is a personal choice. Some people prefer to be tested, to find out what might happen to them and whether anything can be done about it. Others prefer not to be tested as they do not want to carry the psychological burden involved.

Genetics specialists include genetic counsellors, clinical geneticists and cardiologists with expertise in inherited cardiac conditions. The term 'geneticist' is used below and can mean any of these individuals, as appropriate to the stage of your assessment. Geneticists are all trained to work with families and will explain the pros and cons of testing, to help you and your family decide on the choices available to you. They will always respect your decisions on the matter.

How is genetic testing done?

After a referral, and depending on the set-up in each individual centre, you will see the appropriate geneticist. The geneticist will draw up your family tree and ask questions about your medical history and that of each of your family members. They will advise you whether genetic testing would help to find a cause of your dissection and if possible identify any family traits. They will advise whether your family members should also be referred for genetic assessment, which would be a similar process to your own. Family screening would generally apply to your brothers, sisters and children, but if your parents are still alive they should also be included in the assessment.

If your geneticist recommends testing and you agree, you will be asked to sign a consent form and a sample of your blood will be taken for DNA analysis. The sample will be sent away for specialist testing, which often takes up to six months.

How will I receive results?

The geneticist will communicate your results and explain what they mean, either at an appointment, or possibly by letter. If anything is unclear, ask questions until you are satisfied.

You can get three kinds of results from a genetic test.

- A positive result – this is when a genetic change known to be associated with aortic dissection is found in your DNA. This helps doctors decide what the risks are to your health, how to monitor them and how to manage them in the future. At the date of writing, around 30 genetic mutations are known to be associated with aortic dissection, in varying degrees (see the Resources section at the end of this Patient Guide for more detail).

- A negative result – this is when no significant genetic change is found in your DNA. This means either (i) that your dissection did not have a genetic cause, or (ii) that it was not caused by a currently-known gene change. New relevant genetic mutations are being discovered every year.

- A Variant of Unknown clinical Significance (VUS) – this is when a genetic change is found in your DNA but its significance is not clear. It

might be one of the many harmless genetic variations that makes each one of us unique, or it might be the cause of your symptoms. At the moment we just don't know. The clinical geneticist or cardiologist will inform you about what is and is not known about your VUS and may suggest other testing, if appropriate.

Why do family members need imaging?

As you have had an aortic dissection, and even if no known genetic cause can be found, it is common practice for your 'first-degree relatives' (brothers, sisters, children, and parents if still alive) to have an 'imaging' scan of their aorta, to check whether they are at risk.

If you have received a positive genetic test result, your family members would be imaged depending on the decisions made around genetic screening.

How does imaging work?

CT or MRI scans are the most accurate methods of imaging and are the only ways of seeing the whole aorta. An echocardiogram of the ascending aorta may be offered as an initial imaging option but echo scans cannot see the whole aorta. It is important to assess the whole of the aorta.

What if my family members are at risk?

The combination of imaging results and genetic testing gives doctors enough information to work out what someone's risk of an aortic dissection is and whether early medical or surgical intervention will help to manage this risk. Sometimes this involves taking medication to protect the aorta and try to slow down any deterioration. Sometimes it involves having planned surgery to replace a part of the aorta, rather than waiting for a dissection to occur.

The decision on having surgery to prevent a possible future problem is approached by comparing the risk of something bad happening (such as an aortic dissection) with the risk of having the surgery. Surgery is generally considered only when the risk of something bad happening is higher than the risk of the surgery itself. This is an important conversation for patients to have with their specialist.

Resources

Web page links quoted were correct at the time of publishing (2022). Updates will be posted on the resources page of our website.

Membership: As an aortic dissection survivor, or the relative of one, you are eligible for FREE life membership of our national patient association, Aortic Dissection Awareness UK & Ireland. Join at: www.aorticdissectionawareness.org

Online support: The patient association also runs the Aortic Dissection Buddies UK & Ireland Group: www.facebook.com/groups/AorticDissectionUKBuddies.

This Facebook Group is private. Bona fide members who have been affected by aortic dissection can join, post, and view others' posts.

Online information: The internet has many resources available on aortic dissection. One authoritative source designed specifically for those who have suffered an aortic dissection is the IRAD (International Registry of Aortic Dissection) site: livingwithdissection.iradonline.org

A number of abbreviations and acronyms are used in aortic medicine. Aortic Hope in the USA publishes an excellent glossary: www.aortichope.org/post/glossary-of-thoracic-aortic-conditions

Diet: A number of online or physical resources are available which will give you good guidance on a healthy diet. Always use reliable sources such as NHS websites. British Heart Foundation booklets are also good – these can be found online or in any cardiology department or cardiac rehab class.

Exercise: Activity Recommendations for Post-aortic Dissection Patients www.ahajournals.org/doi/full/10.1161/CIRCULATIONAHA.113.005819

See also the IRAD web site page at livingwithdissection.iradonline.org/physical-information/

Online cardiac rehabilitation courses: BHF, see www.bhf.org.uk/informationsupport/support/cardiac-rehabilitation-at-home

Further cardiac rehabilitation classes: Sometimes called 'Phase 4' classes. These are listed at phase-4.cardiac-rehabilitation.net The nurses from your NHS cardiac rehabilitation class (sometimes called Phase 3 classes) should also know if there is one near you. You should only use a Phase 4 class that is BACPR approved.

Mental Health

PTS and PTSD

Critical Illness, Intensive Care and Post-Traumatic Stress Disorder
www.psychologytools.com/resource/critical-illness-intensive-care-and-post-traumatic-stress-disorder-ptsd/ (free resource)

Progressive relaxation and relaxed breathing

www.psychologytools.com/resource/progressive-muscle-relaxation/
www.psychologytools.com/resource/relaxed-breathing/
(Both free resources by signing up to a free account)

Note: full access to the above tools is usually possible via a CBT therapist.

CBT guidance and workbooks

An excellent guide is 'Reclaim Your Life', by Dr Chris Williams, available via store.llttf.com/product/reclaim-your-life-from-illness-disability-pain-or-fatigue-2nd-edition/

The Australian CCI organisation and website is also well-respected: www.cci.health.wa.gov.au/Resources/Looking-After-Yourself

Counselling registration bodies

There are many professional accreditation and registration bodies in the UK covering different sorts of counselling. The following bodies are likely to be an initial choice, though this list does not give personal recommendations:

CBT is mentioned in this Patient Guide several times. The British Association for Behavioural and Cognitive Psychotherapies (BABCP) is the lead organisation for CBT in the UK and lists BABCP accredited CBT therapists and psychologists www.babcp.com.

For EMDR therapists, check www.emdrassociation.org.uk.

Typically, longer-term therapies would be covered by the British Association for Counselling and Psychotherapy (BACP) www.bacp.co.uk/

Other bodies, including those aimed at a specific country, such as Scotland, are listed at www.counselling-directory.org.uk/accreditation.html#registrationaccreditation

Counsellors accredited by these bodies may work in the NHS and/or in private practice.

Blood pressure

BHF web page and video on taking your blood pressure
www.bhf.org.uk/informationsupport/support/manage-your-b ood-
pressure-at-home#measure

AHA/AMA poster with seven tips on how to take an accurate blood
pressure reading:
www.targetbp.org/tools_downloads/mbp/?media_dl=1066

Blood pressure monitors: BHF guidance at
www.bhf.org.uk/informationsupport/heart-matters-magazine/medical/
tests/blood-pressure-measuring-at-home

Warfarin

NICE guidelines on warfarin management are available a-
cks.nice.org.uk/topics/anticoagulation-oral/management/warfarin/

Home monitoring is discussed at
www.nice.org.uk/guidance/dg14/chapter/1-Recommenda-ions

Dental work

Antibiotic protection for dental and other work: NICE Guicance CG64
www.nice.org.uk/guidance/cg64 applies, plus the Scottish Dental CEP
Implementation Advice on CG64, which clarifies CG64 -
www.sdcep.org.uk/published-guidance/antibiotic-prophylaxis/

Genetics

The NHS criteria qualifying you and your relatives for genetic testing can
be found at:

www.england.nhs.uk/wp-content/uploads/2018/08/rare-and-inherited-
disease-eligibility-criteria-v2.pdf

You should refer to section "R125 Thoracic aortic aneurysm or dissection".

Regular updates on genes affecting aortic dissection are published
roughly annually and are listed at www.aorticdissectionawareness.org/
resources.

Notes Pages

Questions to ask your medical carers:

What happened?

What type of aortic dissection did I have?

Can you draw a sketch of what happened that I can keep?

What was my treatment (surgery, medical management?)

Do have any residual dissection?

Did I have a new aortic valve?

Tissue or mechanical?

Did have any other work e.g. a coronary bypass?

How long was I in ICU?

Did have any complications?

Did I suffer ICU delirium?

Can I have a copy of my discharge summary?

What medications do I need?

Which of these are lifelong?

Which can I adjust with my GP?

What are my blood pressure and heart rate targets?

Do I need antibiotics for any dental work?

What are my restrictions on exercise to start with?

When will I be able to drive?

When can I fly?

Space for your own notes

Sketch of your aorta

You᠆ surgeon or consultant can use these diagrams to
draw on (a) what happened to you, and (b) any repair.

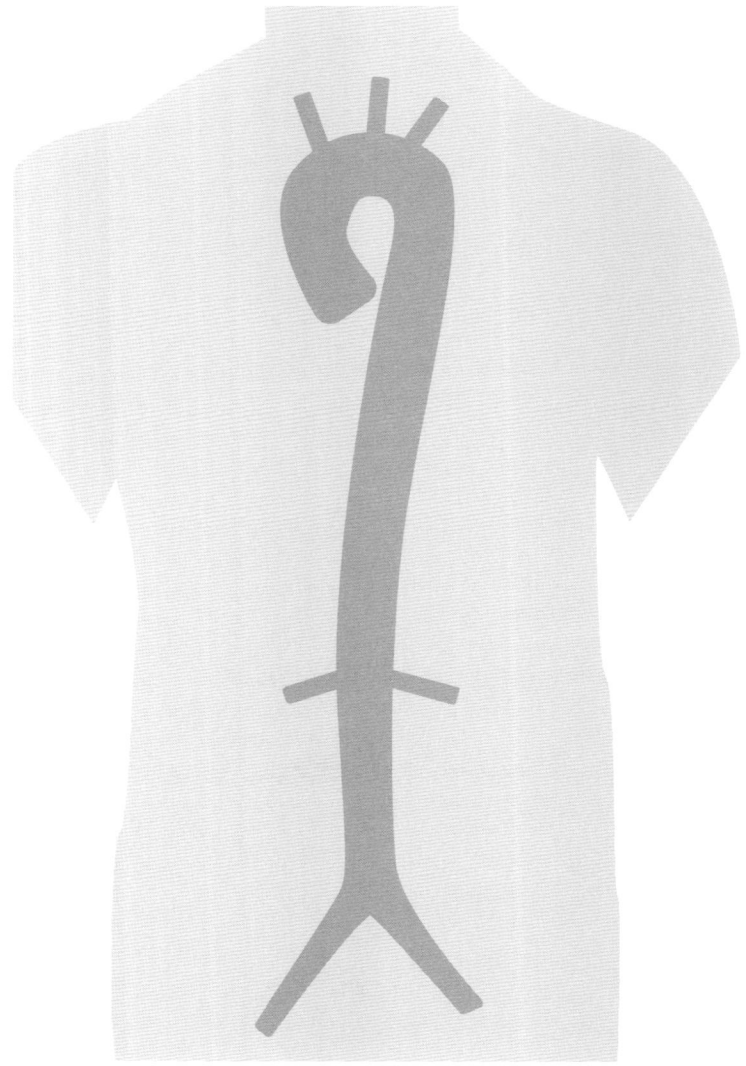

Blank for sketch - extent of dissection of your aorta before treatment

Sketch of your aorta

Your surgeon or consultant can use these diagrams to draw on (a) what happened to you, and (b) any repair.

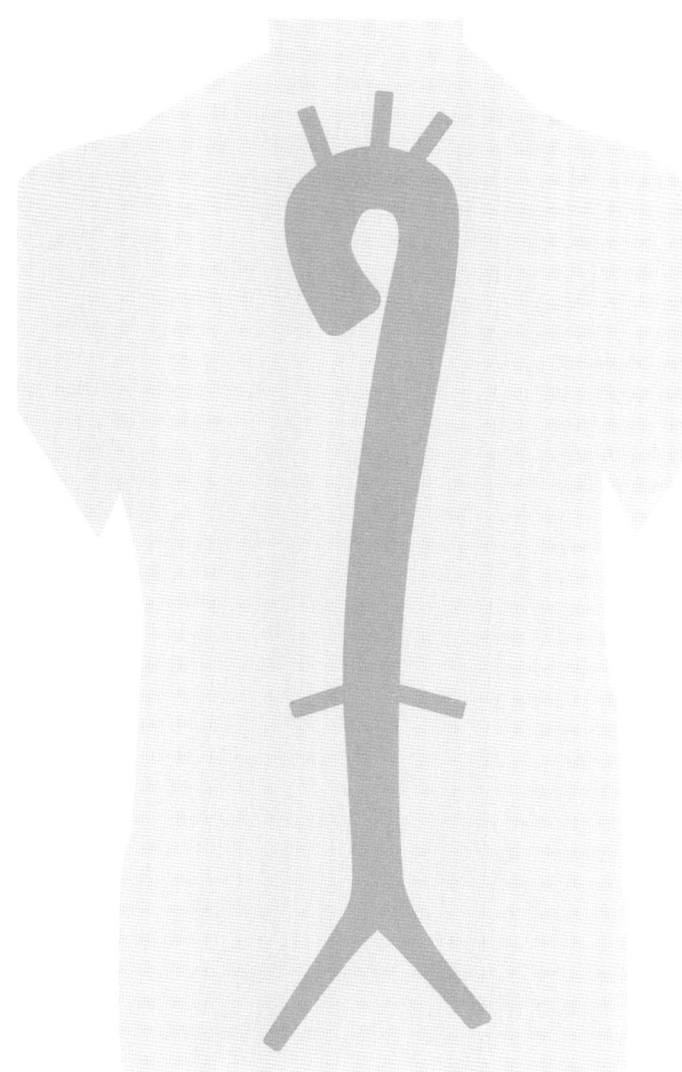

Blank for sketch - Repair or treatment carried out